CORONARY ARTERY DISEASE DIET COOKBOOK FOR NEWLY DIAGNOSED

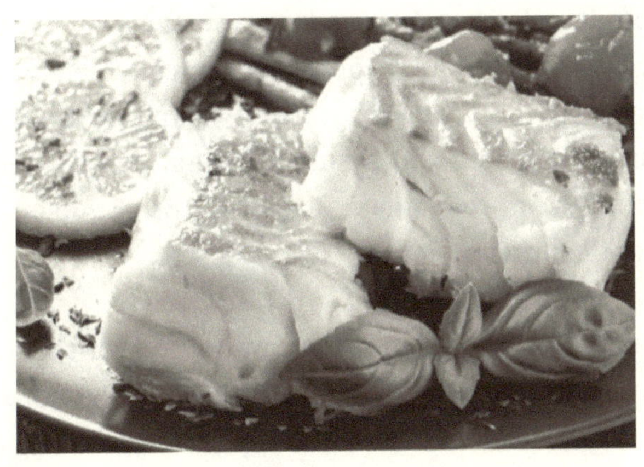

Discover Easy And Flavorful Heart-Healthy Meals For Managing Coronary Artery Disease Without Sacrificing Taste

Kathleen Scribner

TABLE OF CONTENTS

INTRODUCTION

Understanding Coronary Artery Disease (CAD)

Coronary Artery Disease (CAD) is a common cardiovascular ailment that requires sophisticated knowledge to effectively treat. Fundamentally, coronary artery disease (CAD) is caused by the slow buildup of atherosclerotic plaques in the coronary arteries, which obstruct the blood supply to the heart muscle. This illness, which is also known as ischemic heart disease, increases the risk of heart attacks and a number of other cardiovascular problems.

A number of complicated variables interact to cause coronary artery disease (CAD), with atherosclerosis playing a major role. A series of processes are set in motion by atherosclerosis, which is the build-up of inflammatory cells, fatty deposits, and cholesterol within the artery walls. These deposits eventually turn into plaques, which restrict the coronary arteries and reduce the heart's blood flow.

It is essential to comprehend the risk factors linked to CAD for both early intervention and prevention. A sedentary lifestyle, smoking, high blood pressure, diabetes, high cholesterol, and other factors all play a major role in the onset and progression of coronary artery disease (CAD). Genetic predispositions also matter, which highlights the significance of a multifaceted strategy for heart health.

It is essential to identify the signs of CAD in order to take prompt action. Common symptoms include angina (chest pain or discomfort), exhaustion, and irregular heartbeats. ECGs, also known as electrocardiograms, stress tests, and coronary angiography are examples of diagnostic tools that help medical practitioners determine the severity of a patient's disease and create treatment strategies.

A multimodal strategy is used in the care of CAD with the goals of reducing symptoms, averting complications, and improving cardiovascular health in general. The core of CAD management is changing one's lifestyle to include a heart-healthy diet, frequent exercise, and quitting smoking. To reduce risk factors and enhance cardiac function, doctors may give medications including beta-blockers, statins, and antiplatelet medicines.

Interventional treatments such as coronary artery bypass grafting (CABG) or angioplasty with stent implantation may be advised in situations with advanced CAD. These treatments provide hope to patients with significant coronary artery blockages by reducing symptoms and restoring blood flow to the heart muscle.

In order to combat CAD, prevention education is essential. The occurrence and development of CAD can be considerably decreased by highlighting the need of regular health examinations, early risk factor identification, and proactive lifestyle modifications. Promoting heart-healthy eating, consistent exercise, and stress reduction cultivates a proactive cardiovascular health strategy.

Finally, raising awareness and encouraging proactive heart health require an understanding of Coronary Artery Disease. Through an understanding of its pathophysiology, identification of risk factors, and adoption of preventative interventions, people may take control of their cardiovascular health and make educated decisions. This information supports the continuous efforts to lessen the impact of CAD on global health and forms the basis of a heart-healthy lifestyle.

Importance of Diet in Managing CAD

When someone is diagnosed with Coronary Artery Disease (CAD), it is imperative that lifestyle decisions be reevaluated, particularly with regard to nutrition. Through the path of Chloe, a strong individual navigating the complications of CAD, let's explore the significance of nutritional choices.

Picture Chloe, a lively woman in her mid-forties, being informed that she has CAD. After experiencing shock and anxiety, Chloe quickly focused her energies on realizing how she might actively support her own wellbeing. This is where a diet high in heart-healthy fats becomes extremely important.

Chloe learned that eating a heart-healthy diet was a great tool for controlling her CAD rather than only about restriction. She started her journey by realizing the need of eating meals high in nutrients in order to lower her cholesterol and keep her blood pressure in a healthy range. The cornerstones of her redesigned food landscape were whole grains, fruits, vegetables, lean meats, and omega-3 fatty acids.

As Chloe investigated the range of foods that may support her heart health, the significance of nutritional density in treating CAD became clear. Antioxidant, fiber, and vitamin-rich diets improved her health overall and prevented atherosclerosis from worsening, which is an important part of managing coronary artery disease (CAD).

Chloe quickly learned that maintaining ideal blood sugar levels and controlling her weight required a careful dietary balance. Her partners in developing a sustainable strategy went beyond strict adherence to nutritional guidelines: portion management and mindful eating.

Chloe found a plethora of mouthwatering and heart-healthy dishes as she set off on her culinary journey. Her meals evolved into a feast of tastes combined with the intention of nourishing her heart, ranging from colorful salads to nutrient-dense smoothies to filling main entrees.

Beyond Chloe's physical health, a heart-healthy diet has an influence. It started to positively impact her everyday decisions and became a catalyst for lifestyle improvements. Her program included regular exercise and stress reduction, which increased the overall effectiveness of CAD therapy.

We saw firsthand the transformational influence of dietary decisions in Chloe's story. A heart-healthy diet becomes more than just a matter of nourishment; it becomes a source of resilience, empowerment, and optimism. Chloe's experience supports the idea that controlling CAD is a chance for a complete lifestyle makeover, with food playing a critical role in feeding the heart and living a full, heart-healthy life.

CHAPTER ONE: DIETARY FUNDAMENTALS FOR CAD

Nutritional Guidelines for Heart Health

It takes a lifetime of dedication to maintain heart health, beginning with thoughtful food selections. A variety of concepts aimed at promoting cardiovascular health are included in nutritional guidelines for heart health. In order to promote a deeper understanding, let's examine the essential elements of these rules.

1. Embrace a Mediterranean-Inspired Diet:

- Give fruits, vegetables, whole grains, and legumes a priority.
- Include heart-healthy fats from nuts, fatty seafood, and olive oil.
- Choose lean foods like fish and chicken and cut out on red meat.

2. Control Sodium Intake:

- Minimize processed meals heavy in salt.
- Instead of using too much salt, add flavor using herbs and spices.
- Be aware of hidden salt in foods from restaurants, stores, and cans.

3. Opt for Heart-Healthy Fats:

- Healthy fats may be found in avocados, nuts, seeds, and fatty fish.
- Opt for unsaturated fats instead of saturated and trans fats.
- Reduce your consumption of fried and processed meals that are high in unhealthy fats.

4. Prioritize Omega-3 Fatty Acids:

- Include fish high in fat, such as trout, salmon, and mackerel, in your diet.
- Take into account plant-based sources such as walnuts, chia seeds, and flaxseeds.
- Omega-3 fatty acids lower inflammation and raise cholesterol, which are two ways they support heart health.

5. Monitor Cholesterol Intake:

- Restrict the amount of cholesterol you ingest from foods such as organ meats and egg yolks.
- Select plant-based protein substitutes and lean proteins.
- Give special attention to meals that reduce LDL ("bad") cholesterol levels.

6. Increase Fiber Intake:

- For fiber, choose fruits, vegetables, whole grains, and legumes.
- Insoluble fiber promotes digestive health, whereas soluble fiber lowers cholesterol.
- For the greatest advantages, try to eat a range of meals high in fiber.

7. Manage Portion Sizes:

- Pay attention to portion management to avoid overindulging.
- Recognize your signs of hunger and fullness, and steer clear of large, high-calorie meals.
- Throughout the day, eating small, well-balanced meals can help control blood sugar levels.

8. Limit Added Sugars:

- Reduce your intake of processed food and sugar-filled beverages.
- Look for hidden sugars on food labels.
- Select natural sweeteners sparingly, such as honey or maple syrup.

9. Stay Hydrated with Water:

- Water is necessary for heart health as well as general wellbeing.
- Avoid overindulging in sugary beverages and coffee.
Staying well hydrated aids in maintaining ideal blood pressure and promotes healthy blood circulation.

10. Consider Dietary Supplements:

- Before using supplements, speak with a medical practitioner.
- Vitamin D, plant sterols, and omega-3 supplements may be good for heart health.
- A healthy diet ought to be supplemented, not substituted, by supplements.

Following these dietary recommendations promotes a heart-healthy way of living. It's crucial to remember that everyone has different nutritional requirements, and speaking with a medical expert or a qualified dietitian can offer tailored advice. People may actively support a heart-healthy lifestyle and the health of their cardiovascular system by making educated dietary choices.

Role of Various Nutrients in CAD Prevention

Understanding the effects of different nutrients on cardiovascular health is crucial for taking a strategic approach to diet in order to prevent coronary artery disease (CAD). Here, we examine the functions of important nutrients in the prevention of CAD, highlighting the significance of a diet rich in variety.

1. Omega-3 Fatty Acids:

- **Role**: Walnuts, flaxseeds, and fatty fish are rich sources of omega-3 fatty acids, which have anti-inflammatory qualities and lower the risk of atherosclerosis.
- **Effect**: Lowers triglyceride levels, encourages normal blood vessel activity, and improves heart health in general.

2. Fiber:

- **Role**: Whole grains, fruits, and vegetables are rich sources of dietary fiber, which helps lower cholesterol and maintain intestinal health.

- **Effect:** Lowers low-density lipoprotein ("bad") cholesterol, stabilizes blood sugar, and supports a thriving gut microbiota.

3. Antioxidants (Vitamins C and E):

- **Role**: As antioxidants, vitamins C and E shield cells from inflammation and oxidative damage.
- **Effect:** Protects blood vessels from harm, lowers the chance of plaque development, and promotes general cardiovascular health.

4. Potassium:

- **Role**: Bananas, oranges, and leafy greens are good sources of potassium, which lowers blood pressure.
- **Effect:** Lowers the burden on the cardiovascular system and promotes healthy blood pressure by balancing salt levels.

5. Magnesium:

- **Role***:* The function of muscles and nerves, particularly the heart muscle, depends critically on magnesium.
- **Effect:** Helps maintain a stable pulse, controls blood pressure, and enhances the stability of the cardiovascular system as a whole.

6. Plant Sterols:

- **Role**: Plant sterols, which are found in nuts, seeds, and vegetable oils by nature, act as a cholesterol substitute and reduce LDL cholesterol levels.
- **Effect**: Lessens the absorption of cholesterol, promoting a better lipid profile.

7. Coenzyme Q10 (CoQ10):

- **Role:** Heart cells, like all other cells, need CoQ10 to produce energy.
- **Effect:** Helps the heart work better overall, which may lower the chance of developing heart disease.

8. Vitamin D:

- **Role:** The absorption of calcium and bone health depend on vitamin D, which has an indirect effect on cardiovascular health.
- **Effect:** Keeps blood pressure at its ideal level, boosts immunity, and may help avoid heart disease.

9. Potent Phytochemicals:

- **Role:** Phytochemicals, which may be found in vibrant fruits and vegetables, provide protection against a number of illnesses, including heart disease.
- **Effect:** Has anti-inflammatory and antioxidant properties that promote cardiovascular health in general.

10. B Vitamins (B6, B12, Folate):

- Role: The metabolism of homocysteine, an amino acid that is associated with heart disease when it is high, is influenced by B vitamins.

- Effect: Lowers the risk of cardiovascular events and atherosclerosis by maintaining appropriate homocysteine levels.

Including a wide variety of foods high in nutrients in the diet guarantees a holistic approach to the prevention of CAD. The synergistic benefits of these nutrients must be emphasized, underscoring the significance of a diverse and balanced diet for the best possible cardiovascular health. As with any dietary adjustments, seeking the advice of medical specialists or trained dietitians can offer tailored advice depending on a person's unique health requirements and conditions.

Portion Control and Balanced Eating

In the journey to manage Coronary Artery Disease (CAD) and promote overall heart health, mastering portion control and embracing balanced eating becomes paramount. Let's explore how these principles, detailed in our book, serve as the cornerstones of a vibrant and heart-conscious lifestyle.

Understanding Portion Control

Effective portion control is not about deprivation but about making mindful choices regarding the amount of food consumed. It involves being aware of serving sizes and listening to one's body signals of hunger and fullness. In the context of our book, we guide readers on practical strategies to manage portion sizes, fostering a healthier relationship with food.

Strategies for Portion Control

- **Visual Guides**: Introduce visual cues to estimate portion sizes, such as using your hand or everyday objects as a reference.
- **Plate Composition**: Encourage a balanced plate with portions of lean proteins, whole grains, and

colorful vegetables, ensuring a well-rounded and satisfying meal.

- **Mindful Eating**: Promote awareness during meals by savoring each bite, chewing slowly, and recognizing satiety cues, which helps prevent overeating.

Balanced Eating for Heart Health

The secret to giving the body the nutrition it needs to perform at its best is to eat a balanced diet. Our book promotes a balanced dietary strategy that places an emphasis on nutrient-dense foods and restricts excessive consumption of refined carbohydrates, salt, and saturated fats in the context of CAD prevention.

Elements of a Balanced Diet:

- **Diverse Nutrient Sources**: To guarantee an adequate supply of vital nutrients, promote the consumption of a wide variety of fruits, vegetables, whole grains, lean proteins, and healthy fats.
- **Moderation of Unhealthy Choices**: To preserve overall nutritional balance, emphasize moderation

while allowing for flexibility by including occasional treats.

- **Hydration**: Stress the need of drinking enough water for good health as it promotes the health of the heart among other body systems.

Making wholesome food choices and managing portion sizes may be difficult, particularly in the fast-paced world of today. Our book offers helpful advice and methods for overcoming typical challenges like time restraints, emotional eating, and outside factors that might affect dietary decisions.

Beyond specific meals, portion management and balanced eating are essential components of a heart-healthy lifestyle. Our book offers readers step-by-step instructions on how to incorporate these practices into their everyday lives and create long-lasting adjustments that support long-term cardiovascular health.

Our book's emphasis on portion control and balanced eating not only provides readers with useful skills for controlling CAD, but it also promotes a healthy and pleasurable relationship with food. The intention is to provide people the tools they need to make wise decisions, enjoy healthful foods, and develop a lifestyle that complements their path toward heart health.

CHAPTER TWO: THE SCIENCE BEHIND THE RECIPES

Explaining Heart-Healthy Ingredients

In our book, we explore the complex web of heart-healthy components and shed light on how they might be used to treat Coronary Artery Disease (CAD) and improve cardiovascular health. Let's examine the nutrient-dense treasures that are described in our pages to provide readers with knowledge about the components of a diet that is heart-healthy.

1. Fatty Fish: Trout, salmon, and mackerel which are high in omega-3 fatty acids, are essential for lowering the risk of CAD, promoting healthy blood vessel function, and decreasing inflammation.

2. Olive Oil: Extra Virgin Olive Oil is a mainstay of the Mediterranean diet and is rich in antioxidants and monounsaturated fats that help to decrease cholesterol and promote heart health in general.

3. Nuts and Seeds: Chia seeds, flaxseeds, almonds, and walnuts These nuts and seeds, which are rich in fiber, antioxidants, and omega-3 fatty acids, offer a heart-healthy combo that lowers cholesterol and promotes heart health.

4. Whole Grains: Oats, Brown Rice, Quinoa Whole grains, which are high in fiber, support cardiovascular health by stabilizing blood sugar, lowering cholesterol, and improving overall blood pressure.

5. Vibrant Fruits and Vegetables: Bell peppers, spinach, kale, and berries Rich in vitamins, minerals, and antioxidants, these colorful options promote general well-being and lower inflammation, which is good for the heart.

6. Avocado:

- High in Monounsaturated Fats: Avocados are a good source of monounsaturated fats, which can help decrease bad cholesterol and improve lipid profiles.

7. Legumes and Beans:

- **Black beans, lentils, and chickpeas**: Legumes, which are high in fiber and plant-based proteins, help to regulate blood pressure and help with weight loss, both of which promote heart health.

8. Oatmeal

- **Beta-Glucans**: A soluble fiber that lowers cholesterol and promotes cardiovascular health, beta-glucans are found in oats.

9. Garlic:

- **Allicin**: This sulfur-containing ingredient in garlic has been linked to a number of heart-protective advantages, including decreasing cholesterol and blood pressure.

10. Dark Chocolate:

- **Flavanols**: When consumed in moderation, dark chocolate with a high cocoa content has flavonoids, which may improve blood flow and lower blood pressure, both of which are beneficial to heart health.

Not only do we highlight these heart-healthy items in our book, but we also offer helpful advice on how to incorporate them into tasty and nourishing meals. The combination of these components creates the foundation of a heart-healthy diet, enabling readers to make decisions that will benefit their cardiovascular health.

Cooking Techniques for Maximum Nutrient Retention

When it comes to the management of Coronary Artery Disease (CAD), cooking is just as important as the ingredients. Our book places a strong emphasis on cooking methods that optimize nutrient retention so that every mouthful supports heart health. Let's examine these methods that follow the guidelines provided in our extensive guide.

1. Steaming:

Technique: Steaming involves cooking food over boiling water, preserving vitamins and minerals that can be lost through other methods.
Benefits: Retains the vibrant colors and nutritional integrity of vegetables, making it an ideal method for heart-healthy meals.

2. Poaching:

Technique: Poaching involves gently simmering food in a liquid, such as broth or water, minimizing nutrient loss.
Benefits: Preserves the natural flavors and nutrients of delicate proteins like fish or poultry, offering a heart-healthy and flavorful outcome.

3. Sautéing:

Technique: Quick cooking over medium-high heat with a small amount of heart-healthy oil.
Benefits: Preserves the integrity of vegetables while adding a golden hue, enhancing flavors without compromising nutrient content.

4. Grilling:

Technique: Grilling imparts a smoky flavor while allowing excess fats to drip away.
Benefits: Suitable for lean proteins like fish and chicken, preserving their nutritional value while enhancing taste.

5. Baking and Roasting:

Technique: Cooking food in an oven with dry heat, often without added fats.
Benefits: Retains the natural moisture of food while developing robust flavors, suitable for vegetables, lean meats, and whole grains.

6. Blanching:

Technique: Briefly immersing vegetables in boiling water, followed by rapid cooling.
Benefits: Preserves color, texture, and nutrients, making it an effective method for vegetables like broccoli and green beans.

7. Slow Cooking:

Technique: Long, low-temperature cooking in a slow cooker or crockpot.

Benefits: Ideal for tough cuts of meat and legumes, slow cooking enhances flavors and retains nutrients without the need for excessive added fats.

8. Microwaving:

Technique: Quick cooking using microwave radiation.

Benefits: Minimizes nutrient loss due to short cooking times, making it a convenient option for preserving the nutritional value of vegetables.

9. Raw Preparations:

Technique: Consuming certain foods in their raw state.

Benefits: Particularly applicable to fruits, vegetables, and nuts, preserving the maximum nutritional content, especially heat-sensitive vitamins.

10. Stir-Frying:

Technique: Quick cooking with small amounts of oil over high heat.

Benefits: Preserves the color, texture, and nutritional value of vegetables and lean proteins, offering a flavorful and heart-healthy option.

In our book, we walk readers through the process of incorporating these cooking methods into their repertoire so that preparing heart-healthy food is as enjoyable as it is nutritious. By using these strategies, people may enjoy wholesome and tasty meals that support cardiovascular health and aid in the overall treatment of CAD.

CHAPTER THREE: DELICIOUS AND NUTRITIOUS BREAKFASTS

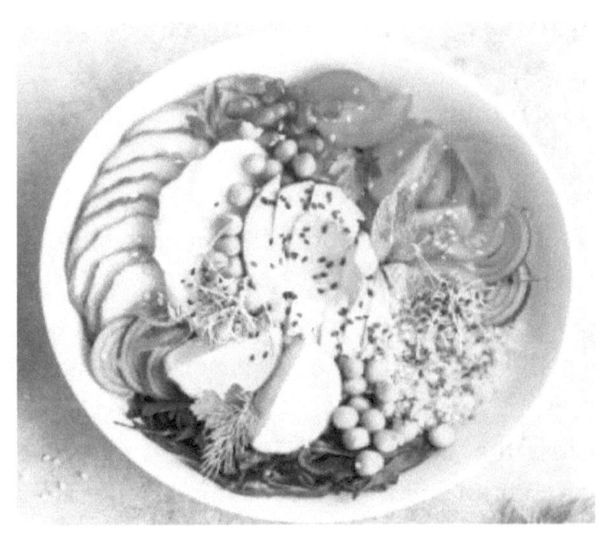

1. Apple Cinnamon Overnight Oats

Ingredients:

- 1/2 cup rolled oats
- 1/2 cup unsweetened almond milk (or any preferred milk)
- 1/2 apple, grated or finely chopped
- 1 tablespoon chia seeds
- 1/2 teaspoon ground cinnamon
- 1/2 teaspoon vanilla extract
- **Optional:** a drizzle of honey or maple syrup for sweetness

Instructions:

1. Place rolled oats, unsweetened almond milk, diced or shredded apple, chia seeds, ground cinnamon, and vanilla essence in a jar or container.
2. To guarantee a uniform distribution, thoroughly stir the components.
3. Depending on your preference, you can optionally add a drizzle of honey or maple syrup for sweetness.
4. Close the jar or container and let it in the fridge for the entire night so the flavors and fluids may seep into the oats.
5. Give the Apple Cinnamon Overnight Oats a thorough toss in the morning.
6. For added taste and freshness, top with more apple slices or a dusting of cinnamon, if preferred.

7. Savor this tasty and easy breakfast choice that is full of heart-healthy nutrients and fiber.

2. Smoked Salmon and Cream Cheese Bagel

Ingredients:

- 1 whole grain bagel, sliced and toasted
- Light cream cheese
- Smoked salmon
- Sliced cucumber and tomato

Instructions:

1. Toast the whole grain bagel until it reaches the crispiness you like.
2. Top each half of the toasted bagel with a layer of light cream cheese.
3. Place smoked salmon slices over the cream cheese.
4. To add freshness and crunch to the smoked salmon, thinly slice a tomato and cucumber over it.
5. For extra taste, you may optionally add a squeeze of lemon juice or a sprinkling of fresh dill.
6. To make a sandwich, place the second half of the bagel on top.

7. Present the Bagel with Smoked Salmon and Cream Cheese right away, and enjoy a delicious and heart-healthy brunch or breakfast.

3. Sweet Potato and Black Bean Breakfast Burrito

Ingredients:

- 1 large sweet potato, peeled and diced
- 1 can black beans, drained and rinsed
- 4 large eggs, scrambled
- Whole wheat or corn tortillas
- Avocado slices
- Salsa
- Fresh cilantro, chopped
- Olive oil for cooking
- Salt and pepper to taste

Instructions:

1. Heat the olive oil in a skillet over medium heat. Sweet potatoes should be added and sautéed until they are soft and start to caramelize.
2. Cook the sweet potatoes and drained black beans in a pan until they are well cooked.

3. Scramble the eggs in a different pan until they are cooked through. Add pepper and salt for seasoning.

4. Use a dry skillet or the microwave to reheat the tortillas.

5. Place some of the sweet potato and black bean mixture onto a tortilla to assemble the breakfast burritos.

6. Top with a few avocado slices, salsa, scrambled eggs, and fresh cilantro.

7. To make a burrito, fold the tortilla's edges inward and roll it up.

8. Continue with the leftover tortillas.

9. Enjoy a tasty, high-protein meal by serving the Sweet Potato and Black Bean meal Burrito right away.

4. Pineapple Coconut Chia Pudding

Ingredients:

- 1 cup coconut milk
- 1/2 cup diced pineapple
- 1/4 cup chia seeds
- 1 tablespoon honey or maple syrup (optional, for sweetness)
- 1/4 teaspoon vanilla extract (optional)

Instructions:

1. Place the chopped pineapple, chia seeds, coconut milk, honey (or maple syrup, if desired), and vanilla extract (if desired) in a mixing bowl. To equally mix all components, give it a good stir.
2. To enable the chia seeds to soak up the liquid and thicken, cover the bowl and place it in the refrigerator for at least two hours, or better yet, overnight.
3. After the mixture has cooled, thoroughly stir it to make sure all of the chia seeds have dissolved into a pudding-like consistency.
4. You may serve the chilled pineapple coconut chia pudding alone or, if you'd like, sprinkle with more chopped pineapple, shredded coconut, or a honey drizzle.

5. *Almond Flour Pancakes with Fresh Berries*

Ingredients:

- 1 cup almond flour
- 2 tablespoons coconut flour
- 1 teaspoon baking powder
- 1/4 teaspoon salt
- 2 large eggs

- 1/2 cup unsweetened almond milk (or any preferred milk)
- 1 tablespoon maple syrup (optional)
- 1 teaspoon vanilla extract
- Fresh berries for topping (e.g., blueberries, strawberries)

Instructions:

1. Combine the almond flour, coconut flour, baking powder, and salt in a bowl.
2. Beat the eggs in another dish and stir in the almond milk, vanilla extract, and maple syrup (if using). Blend well.
3. Mix the dry and wet ingredients together, stirring gently until blended. To thicken, let the batter sit for a few minutes.
4. Turn up the heat to medium on a nonstick skillet or griddle.
5. Transfer the mixture onto the skillet to create pancakes with the size you want.
6. Cook the pancakes until bubbles appear on their surface, then turn them over and cook the second side until it turns golden brown.
7. Continue cooking the pancakes until they are all done.
8. Arrange the pancakes in a stack on a platter and cover with an abundance of fresh berries.

9. If desired, add a little maple syrup to the drizzle for sweetness.

10. Present the warm Almond Flour Pancakes with Fresh Berries and savor a filling and delectable morning meal.

6. Veggie and Feta Omelette

Ingredients:

- 3 large eggs
- 1/4 cup diced bell peppers (any color)
- 1/4 cup diced tomatoes
- 1/4 cup diced onion
- 1/4 cup chopped spinach
- 1/4 cup crumbled feta cheese
- Salt and pepper to taste
- 1 tablespoon olive oil or butter

Instructions:

1. Beat the eggs well in a small basin. To taste, add salt and pepper for seasoning.

2. In a nonstick skillet, heat the butter or olive oil over medium heat.

3. Fill the skillet with the chopped tomatoes, onions, and bell peppers. Simmer the veggies for two to three minutes, or until they are tender.

4. Cook the chopped spinach in the pan for a further one to two minutes, or until it wilts.

5. Evenly cover all of the sautéed veggies in the skillet with the beaten eggs by pouring them over them.

6. Leave the eggs in the skillet alone for a few minutes, or until the edges begin to gently peel off the bottom.

7. Evenly distribute the feta cheese crumbles on one half of the omelet.

8. Using a spatula, carefully fold the remaining omelet over the filling to form a half-moon. To seal, lightly press down.

9. Continue cooking for an additional one to two minutes, or until the cheese has melted and the eggs are well cooked.

10. Transfer the omelet to a platter and enjoy it warm.

7. *Whole Grain Waffles with Greek Yogurt and Honey*

Ingredients:

- 1 cup whole wheat flour
- 1/2 cup oats (quick or rolled)
- 2 teaspoons baking powder
- 1/4 teaspoon salt
- 1 tablespoon honey or maple syrup
- 1 cup milk (dairy or plant-based)
- 1/4 cup unsweetened applesauce or mashed banana
- 2 tablespoons melted butter or coconut oil
- 1 teaspoon vanilla extract
- Greek yogurt, for serving
- Honey or maple syrup, for serving
- **Optional toppings:** fresh berries, sliced bananas, chopped nuts

Instructions:

1. As directed by the manufacturer, preheat your waffle iron.
2. Combine the oats, baking powder, whole wheat flour, and salt in a large mixing basin.
3. Combine the milk, melted butter or coconut oil, applesauce or mashed banana, honey or maple syrup, and vanilla extract in another bowl.
4. Add the liquid mixture to the dry mixture and whisk just until incorporated. Take caution not to mix too much.
5. Use cooking spray or melted butter to lightly oil the waffle iron that has been preheated.

6. Evenly distribute the waffle batter in the waffle iron's middle. Once the waffles are golden brown and crispy, follow the manufacturer's directions and cover the pan.

7. After the waffles are done, gently take them out of the waffle pan and place them on serving plates.

8. Top the whole grain waffles with your preferred toppings, such chopped nuts, sliced bananas, or fresh berries, and serve with a dollop of Greek yogurt and a drizzle of honey or maple syrup.

9. Savor these hearty and delectable waffles for a filling brunch or breakfast!

8. Quinoa and Fruit Breakfast Bowl

Ingredients:

- 1/2 cup quinoa, rinsed
- 1 cup water
- 1/2 teaspoon cinnamon
- 1 tablespoon honey or maple syrup (optional, for sweetness)
- 1/2 cup mixed fresh fruits (such as berries, sliced bananas, diced mango, or kiwi)
- 2 tablespoons chopped nuts or seeds (such as almonds, walnuts, or pumpkin seeds)
- 1 tablespoon Greek yogurt (optional, for topping)

Instructions:

1. Place the washed quinoa, water, and cinnamon in a small saucepan. Heat to a boil on a medium-high heat setting.
2. After the quinoa reaches a boiling point, lower the heat to a simmer, cover, and cook for 15 to 20 minutes, or until the water has been absorbed. Using a fork, fluff the quinoa.
3. Add honey or maple syrup, if preferred, to taste.
4. Spoon the cooked quinoa into dishes for dishing.
5. Add chopped nuts or seeds and a variety of fresh fruits on the top of the quinoa.
6. **Optional**: Top with a dollop of Greek yogurt for additional protein and richness.
7. Present the breakfast bowls with quinoa and fruit right away, and relish!

9. Tomato and Basil Avocado Toast

Ingredients:

- 2 slices whole grain bread
- 1 ripe avocado
- 1 medium tomato, sliced
- Fresh basil leaves
- Salt and pepper to taste
- Red pepper flakes (optional, for added spice)

- Lemon juice (optional, for extra flavor)

Instructions:

1. Toast the whole grain bread slices until crispy and golden brown.
2. Use a fork to mash the ripe avocado in a small bowl while the bread is toasting. If preferred, add a squeeze of lemon juice and season with salt and pepper.
3. After the bread is done, equally distribute the mashed avocado over each piece.
4. Place some fresh tomato slices on top of the avocado toast.
5. Tear a few leaves of fresh basil and distribute them on top of the tomato slices.
6. For an extra fiery burst, feel free to top with red pepper flakes.
7. Present the Tomato and Basil Avocado Toast right away, and savor it as a wholesome and delectable alternative for breakfast, brunch, or a snack!

10. Spinach and Mushroom Frittata

Ingredients:

- 6 large eggs

- 1 cup fresh spinach leaves, roughly chopped
- 1 cup mushrooms, sliced
- 1/2 onion, diced
- 1 garlic clove, minced
- 1/2 cup shredded cheese (such as mozzarella, cheddar, or feta)
- 2 tablespoons olive oil
- Salt and pepper to taste

Instructions:

1. Set the oven temperature to 175°C, or 350°F.
2. Whisk the eggs until they are thoroughly beaten in a mixing basin. To taste, add salt and pepper for seasoning. Put aside.
3. In an oven-safe skillet, preheat the olive oil over medium heat.
4. Fill the pan with chopped onion and minced garlic. Simmer the onion for two to three minutes, or until it is aromatic and transparent.
5. Add the sliced mushrooms to the skillet and simmer for 5 to 7 minutes, or until they are softened and golden brown.
6. Cook the chopped spinach in the pan for two minutes, or until it wilts.
7. Evenly distribute the cooked veggies across the skillet.
8. Ensure that the veggies are spread equally by pouring the beaten eggs over them in the skillet.

9. Scatter cheese shredded on top of the frittata.

10. Place the pan in the oven that has been warmed, and bake for 15 to 20 minutes, or until the top of the frittata is gently browned.

11. After the frittata is done, take it out of the oven and allow it to cool somewhat.

12. Cut the frittata into wedges and either serve warm or cold.

11. Cherry Almond Smoothie Bowl

Ingredients:

- 1 cup frozen cherries
- 1 ripe banana, frozen
- 1/2 cup almond milk (or any milk of your choice)
- 1/4 cup Greek yogurt
- 2 tablespoons almond butter
- 1 tablespoon honey or maple syrup (optional, for added sweetness)
- 1 tablespoon chia seeds (optional, for extra fiber and nutrients)
- **Toppings:** sliced almonds, fresh cherries, granola, shredded coconut

Instructions:

1. Put the frozen banana, cherries, almond milk, Greek yogurt, almond butter, chia seeds, honey, or maple syrup (if using) in a blender.
2. Process on high speed until smooth and creamy; adjust consistency with additional almond milk if necessary.
3. Transfer the mixed smoothie into a bowl.
4. You may add whatever kind of toppings you choose to the smoothie bowl, such as sliced almonds, fresh cherries, granola, and shredded coconut.
5. Present your revitalizing and nourishing Cherry Almond Smoothie Bowl right away and relish!

12. Turmeric and Spinach Scrambled Eggs

Ingredients:

- 4 large eggs
- 1 cup fresh spinach leaves, chopped
- 1/2 teaspoon ground turmeric
- 1 tablespoon olive oil or butter
- Salt and pepper to taste
- Optional toppings: diced tomatoes, crumbled feta cheese, chopped fresh herbs

Instructions:

1. Crack the eggs into a mixing dish and whisk until well beaten. Add ground turmeric, salt, and pepper for seasoning. Put aside.

2. In a pan over medium heat, melt butter or olive oil.

3. Cook the chopped spinach in the pan for approximately two minutes, or until it wilts.

4. Add the beaten eggs and wilted spinach to the skillet.

5. Cook the eggs and spinach until they are set and cooked to your preferred consistency, stirring gently with a spatula.

6. After cooking, take the skillet off of the burner.

7. Present the spinach and turmeric scrambled eggs right away, topped with optional extras like chopped fresh herbs, sliced tomatoes, or crumbled feta cheese.

13. Cottage Cheese and Pineapple Parfait

Ingredients:

- 1 cup cottage cheese
- 1 cup diced pineapple (fresh or canned, drained)

- 1/4 cup granola
- 1 tablespoon honey or maple syrup (optional, for added sweetness)
- **Optional toppings:** shredded coconut, chopped nuts, mint leaves

Instructions:

Place half of the cottage cheese in the bottom of a dish or serving glass.
2. Cover the cottage cheese with a layer of chopped pineapple.
3. Scatter granola on top of the pineapple.
4. If wanted, drizzle with more sweetness by using honey or maple syrup.
5. Recreate the layers using the leftover granola, pineapple, and cottage cheese.
6. Garnish the parfait with optional toppings such as chopped nuts, shredded coconut, or mint leaves.
7. Present the cottage cheese and pineapple parfait right away, then savor it!

14. Blueberry Walnut Baked Oatmeal

Ingredients:

- 2 cups old-fashioned oats
- 1/2 cup chopped walnuts

- 1 teaspoon baking powder
- 1/2 teaspoon cinnamon
- 1/4 teaspoon salt
- 2 cups milk (dairy or plant-based)
- 1/3 cup maple syrup
- 1 large egg
- 2 tablespoons melted butter or coconut oil
- 1 teaspoon vanilla extract
- 1 cup fresh or frozen blueberries

Instructions:

1. Adjust the oven temperature to 350°F (175°C) and coat a baking dish with oil.

2. Put the oats, chopped walnuts, baking powder, cinnamon, and salt in a big basin.

3. Combine the milk, egg, maple syrup, melted butter or coconut oil, and vanilla extract in a separate dish.

4. Add the liquid components to the dry ingredients and stir well.

5. Fold the blueberries in gently.

6. Evenly distribute the mixture throughout the baking dish after pouring it in.

7. Bake for 30 to 35 minutes, or until the oatmeal is set and the top is golden brown, in a preheated oven.

8. Before serving, let it cool for a few minutes. Optionally top with a dollop of yogurt or more maple syrup drizzle.

15. *Avocado and Tomato Breakfast Wrap*

Ingredients:

- 1 large whole-grain tortilla
- 1 ripe avocado, sliced
- 1 medium tomato, sliced
- 2 eggs, scrambled
- Salt and pepper to taste
- **Optional**: Salsa or hot sauce for extra flavor
- **Optional**: Fresh cilantro or chopped green onions for garnish

Instructions:

1. Scramble the eggs in a pan over medium heat until they are done to your preference. Add pepper and salt for seasoning.
2. To make the whole-grain tortilla malleable, warm it briefly in the skillet or microwave.

3. Transfer the heated tortilla to a level surface. Arrange the tomato and avocado slices in the middle of the tortilla.

4. Place a spoonful of the scrambled eggs over the tomato and avocado.

5. For added taste, if preferred, add salsa or spicy sauce.

6. To make a wrap, fold the tortilla in half on the edges and roll it up from the bottom.

7. You can choose to add chopped green onions or fresh cilantro as a garnish.

8. Present your Avocado and Tomato Breakfast Wrap right away and savor it!

16. *Peach and Raspberry Yogurt Parfait*

Ingredients:

- 1 cup Greek yogurt (plain or vanilla)
- 1 ripe peach, diced
- 1/2 cup fresh raspberries
- 1/4 cup granola
- 1 tablespoon honey or maple syrup (optional, for added sweetness)
- **Optional toppings:** sliced almonds, shredded coconut, mint leaves

Instructions:

1. To begin, place a tablespoon of Greek yogurt in the bottom of a serving glass or dish.
2. Cover the yogurt with a layer of chopped peaches.
3. Top the peaches with a few fresh raspberries.
4. Add granola on top for some crunch and texture.
5. Continue layering until the glass or bowl is full; add one more layer of Greek yogurt on top to complete.
6. If preferred, drizzle with honey or maple syrup for extra sweetness.
7. For a decorative touch, top the parfait with optional garnishes like sliced almonds, shredded coconut, or mint leaves.
8. Present the Yogurt Parfait with Peaches and Raspberry right away, then relish!

17. Sunflower Seed Butter and Banana Sandwich

Ingredients:

- 2 slices of whole-grain bread
- Sunflower seed butter

- 1 ripe banana, sliced
- Honey (optional)

Instructions:

1. On one side of every bread piece, generously spread sunflower seed butter.
2. Evenly distribute banana slices on one piece of bread.
3. For extra sweetness, you may want to sprinkle honey over the banana slices.
4. Top the slice covered in banana with the remaining piece of bread, butter side down.
5. Gently press the sandwich together.
6. To make handling the sandwich easier, you might choose to cut it in half.

18. *Mango Tango Chia Seed Smoothie*

Ingredients:

- 1 cup frozen mango chunks
- 1 ripe banana, frozen
- 1 cup coconut water or almond milk
- 2 tablespoons chia seeds

- 1 tablespoon honey or maple syrup (optional, for added sweetness)
- Juice of 1 lime (optional, for extra tanginess)
- Ice cubes (optional, for a colder smoothie)

Instructions:

1. Place the frozen banana and mango chunks, chia seeds, coconut water or almond milk, honey or maple syrup (if desired), and lime juice (if desired) in a blender.
2. For a cooler smoothie, feel free to add a few ice cubes.
3. Process on high speed until smooth and creamy; if necessary, add extra liquid to get the right consistency.
4. After blending, taste the smoothie and add extra honey, maple syrup, or lime juice as necessary to modify the sweetness or tanginess.
5. Immediately serve the Mango Tango Chia Seed Smoothie by pouring it into glasses.

19. Egg White Breakfast Burrito with Salsa

Ingredients:

- 1 large whole-grain or spinach tortilla
- 1 cup egg whites (equivalent to about 4-6 large egg whites)
- Salt and pepper to taste
- 1/4 cup diced bell peppers (any color)
- 1/4 cup diced onions
- 1/4 cup shredded cheese (cheddar, Monterey Jack, or your choice)
- Salsa for topping
- **Optional**: Fresh cilantro or sliced avocado for garnish

Instructions:

1. Saute chopped onions and bell peppers in a nonstick pan over medium heat until they are soft.
2. Transfer the egg whites to the skillet, add salt and pepper to taste, and scramble the eggs until they are cooked through.
3. To make the tortilla malleable, warm it briefly in a pan or microwave.
4. In the center of the tortilla, place the cooked egg whites.
5. While the egg whites are still warm, scatter the grated cheese on top to gently melt it.
6. For added taste, feel free to add sliced avocado or fresh cilantro.
7. To form a burrito, fold in the tortilla's sides and roll it up from the bottom.

8. Add your preferred salsa on top.

20. Coconut and Berry Quinoa Porridge

Ingredients:

- 1/2 cup quinoa, rinsed
- 1 cup coconut milk
- 1/2 cup water
- 2 tablespoons shredded coconut (unsweetened)
- 1 tablespoon maple syrup or honey
- 1/2 teaspoon vanilla extract
- Pinch of salt
- Mixed berries (strawberries, blueberries, raspberries) for topping
- **Optional**: Chopped nuts (almonds, walnuts) for garnish

Instructions:

1. Make sure to rinse the quinoa with cool water.
2. Place the rinsed quinoa, water, shredded coconut, vanilla essence, maple syrup or honey, and a little amount of salt in a pot.
3. After bringing the mixture to a boil, turn down the heat. For fifteen to twenty minutes, or until the

quinoa is cooked and the liquid has been absorbed, cover and simmer.

4. To ensure uniform cooking and avoid sticking, stir from time to time.

5. Using a fork, fluff the cooked quinoa.

6. Ladle the quinoa porridge into dishes and garnish with chopped nuts if desired and mixed berries.

7. If preferred, drizzle with more honey or maple syrup.

CHAPTER FOUR: HEART-HEALTHY LUNCHES

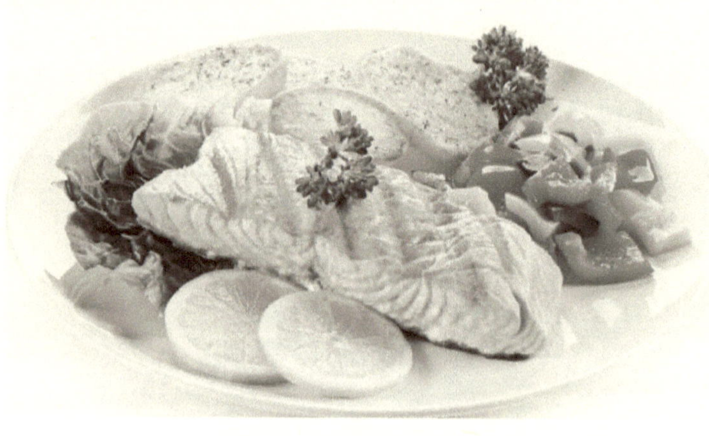

1. Grilled Chicken Salad with Mixed Greens

Ingredients:

- 2 boneless, skinless chicken breasts

- 6 cups mixed salad greens (such as lettuce, spinach, arugula)
- 1 cup cherry tomatoes, halved
- 1/2 cucumber, sliced
- 1/4 red onion, thinly sliced
- 1/4 cup crumbled feta cheese
- 1/4 cup sliced almonds
- Salt and pepper to taste
- Olive oil for grilling

For the Marinade:

- 2 tablespoons olive oil
- 2 cloves garlic, minced
- 1 teaspoon dried oregano
- 1 teaspoon dried thyme
- Juice of 1 lemon
- Salt and pepper to taste

For the Dressing:

- 3 tablespoons extra virgin olive oil
- 2 tablespoons balsamic vinegar
- 1 teaspoon Dijon mustard
- 1 teaspoon honey
- Salt and pepper to taste

Instructions:

1. Combine the marinade ingredients in a small bowl, whisking in the lemon juice, olive oil, minced garlic, dried oregano, dried thyme, salt, and pepper.

2. Transfer the chicken breasts to a shallow dish or plastic bag that can be sealed, and cover them with the marinade. Make sure the chicken has a good coating. Refrigerate for a minimum of 30 minutes or for up to 4 hours after covering or sealing.

3. Set the grill's temperature to medium-high. To keep the grill grates from sticking, lightly grease them with olive oil.

4. Take out the marinated chicken breasts and throw away any extra marinade. Add salt and pepper to the chicken to season it.

5. Place the chicken breasts on the grill and cook for 6 to 8 minutes on each side, or until the internal temperature reaches 165°F (75°C). Before slicing, take them from the grill and give them some time to rest.

6. Prepare the salad ingredients while the chicken is roasting. Combine the mixed salad greens, sliced almonds, cucumber, red onion, crumbled feta cheese, and cherry tomatoes in a big bowl.

7. Combine the extra virgin olive oil, balsamic vinegar, Dijon mustard, honey, salt, and pepper in a small bowl to make the dressing.

8. After the chicken has rested, finely slice it.

9. Distribute the mixed greens and additional ingredients among serving dishes to make the salad.

Add some grilled chicken pieces on the top of each salad.

10. Cover the salads with a drizzle of balsamic vinaigrette dressing.

11. Present the grilled chicken salad right away with mixed greens, and dig in!

2. Salmon and Quinoa Stuffed Bell Peppers

Ingredients:

- 4 large bell peppers (any color)
- 1 cup cooked quinoa
- 2 cans (about 14 oz each) canned salmon, drained
- 1 cup cherry tomatoes, halved
- 1/2 cup feta cheese, crumbled
- 1/4 cup red onion, finely chopped
- 2 cloves garlic, minced
- 2 tablespoons fresh dill, chopped
- 1 tablespoon lemon juice
- 2 tablespoons olive oil
- Salt and pepper to taste

Instructions:

1. Turn the oven on to 375°F, or 190°C.

2. Remove the bell peppers' membranes and seeds by cutting off their tops.
3. Combine cooked quinoa, cherry tomatoes, feta cheese, minced garlic, fresh dill, lemon juice, olive oil, and drained canned salmon in a large mixing dish. Blend well.
4. To taste, add salt and pepper to the mixture.
5. Stuff the salmon and quinoa mixture into each bell pepper.
6. Transfer the filled bell peppers to an oven proof tray.
7. Bake the peppers for 25 to 30 minutes, or until they are soft, in a preheated oven.
8. Before serving, you can choose to add more fresh dill as a garnish.

3. Vegetarian Lentil Soup with Whole Grain Roll

Ingredients:

For the Lentil Soup:

- 1 cup dried green or brown lentils, rinsed
- 1 onion, diced
- 2 carrots, diced
- 2 celery stalks, diced

- 2 cloves garlic, minced
- 6 cups vegetable broth
- 1 can (14 oz) diced tomatoes
- 1 teaspoon ground cumin
- 1 teaspoon ground coriander
- 1/2 teaspoon smoked paprika
- Salt and pepper to taste
- 2 tablespoons olive oil
- Fresh parsley or cilantro for garnish (optional)

For the Whole Grain Rolls:

- 2 cups whole wheat flour
- 1 cup warm water
- 1 tablespoon honey or maple syrup
- 1 packet (2 1/4 teaspoons) active dry yeast
- 1 teaspoon salt
- 1 tablespoon olive oil

Instructions:

For the Lentil Soup:

1. In a large saucepan over medium heat, warm the olive oil. Add the celery, carrots, and chopped onion. Simmer the veggies for 5 minutes or until they are tender.

2. Add the smoked paprika, minced garlic, ground cumin, ground coriander, salt, and pepper. Once fragrant, stir and cook for an additional minute.

3. Fill the saucepan with the chopped tomatoes (with their juices), vegetable broth, and washed lentils. Once the lentils are soft, decrease the heat to low and simmer for 20 to 25 minutes after bringing to a boil.

4. Taste and, if necessary, adjust seasoning. If the soup gets too thick, add extra water or broth.

5. Garnish the hot vegetarian lentil soup with cilantro or fresh parsley, if preferred.

For the Whole Grain Rolls:

1. Dissolve honey or maple syrup in warm water in a large mixing dish. After adding the yeast to the water, let it rest for five to ten minutes, or until frothy.

2. Fill the basin with salt and whole wheat flour. Stir to make a dough.

3. Using a floured surface, knead the dough for approximately five minutes, or until it becomes elastic and smooth.

4. Transfer the dough to a basin that has been gently oiled, cover it with a fresh cloth, and let it rest in a warm location until it has doubled in size, approximately an hour.

5. Turn the oven on to 375°F, or 190°C. The rising dough should be pounded down and divided into six equal parts. Roll each part into a ball and arrange on a parchment paper-lined baking sheet.

6. Apply a little layer of olive oil to the rolls' tops. Bake for 15 to 20 minutes, or until the rolls are golden brown, in a preheated oven.

7. Present the vegetarian lentil soup with the warm whole grain rolls on the side.

4. Mushroom and Spinach Whole Wheat Pizza

Ingredients:

- 1 whole wheat pizza crust (store-bought or homemade)
- 1/2 cup pizza sauce
- 1 1/2 cups shredded mozzarella cheese
- 1 cup sliced mushrooms
- 2 cups fresh spinach leaves, washed and dried
- 1/2 red onion, thinly sliced
- 2 cloves garlic, minced
- 1 tablespoon olive oil
- Salt and pepper to taste
- Crushed red pepper flakes (optional for added spice)

Instructions:

1. Preheat your oven to 425°F (220°C) or as directed on the pizza crust package.
2. Roll out your handmade dough onto a baking sheet or pizza stone if you're using one.
3. Evenly cover the crust with pizza sauce, leaving a thin border all the way around.
4. Top the sauce with mozzarella cheese that has been shredded.
5. Heat the olive oil in a pan over medium heat. Add the minced garlic, red onion, and sliced mushrooms. Sauté the mushrooms until they become soft.
6. Cook the fresh spinach in the pan until it wilts little. Add pepper and salt for seasoning.
7. Evenly distribute the sautéed spinach and mushroom combination over the pizza's cheese.
8. Bake for 12 to 15 minutes in a preheated oven, or until the cheese is bubbling and melted and the crust is brown.
9. For added spiciness, you can optionally top with crushed red pepper flakes.

5. Baked Cod with Lemon-Dill Sauce

Ingredients:

For the Baked Cod:

- 4 cod filets (about 6 oz each)
- 2 tablespoons olive oil
- Salt and pepper to taste
- 2 cloves garlic, minced
- 1 lemon, sliced
- Fresh dill sprigs for garnish

For the Lemon-Dill Sauce:

- 1/2 cup Greek yogurt
- 1 tablespoon fresh lemon juice
- 1 tablespoon chopped fresh dill
- 1 teaspoon Dijon mustard
- Salt and pepper to taste

Instructions:

For the Baked Cod:

1. Turn the oven on to 375°F, or 190°C. Apply a thin layer of olive oil or nonstick cooking spray to a baking dish.
2. Using paper towels, pat the cod filets dry before placing them in the baking dish that has been ready.

3. Cover the cod filets with a drizzle of olive oil. Rub the fish evenly with a mixture of salt, pepper, and chopped garlic for flavor.
4. Top each cod filet with a slice of lemon.
5. Bake for 15 to 20 minutes, or until a fork can easily pierce the fish, in a preheated oven.
6. Make the Lemon-Dill Sauce while the cod bakes.

For the Lemon-Dill Sauce:

1. In a small bowl, use a whisk to thoroughly mix and blend the Greek yogurt, Dijon mustard, chopped dill, fresh lemon juice, salt, and pepper.
2. If necessary, taste and adjust the seasoning.

To Serve:

1. After the cod is done, take it out of the oven and give it some time to rest.
2. Drizzle the hot baked cod filets with the Lemon-Dill Sauce.
3. Add fresh dill sprigs as a garnish.
4. Serve with your preferred side dishes, like a green salad, roasted potatoes, or steamed veggies.

6. Chickpea and Vegetable Stir-Fry

Ingredients:

- 1 can (15 oz) chickpeas, drained and rinsed
- 2 cups mixed vegetables (broccoli, bell peppers, snap peas, carrots, etc.), chopped
- 1 tablespoon sesame oil or vegetable oil
- 3 cloves garlic, minced
- 1 tablespoon ginger, grated
- 2 tablespoons soy sauce
- 1 tablespoon hoisin sauce
- 1 teaspoon rice vinegar
- 1 teaspoon sesame seeds (optional)
- Green onions, sliced for garnish (optional)
- Cooked brown rice or quinoa for serving

Instructions:

1. Heat the sesame oil in a big pan or wok over medium-high heat.
2. Sauté the grated ginger and chopped garlic in the heated oil for about 30 seconds, or until fragrant.
3. Stir-fry the mixed veggies in the skillet for three to five minutes, or until they start to get tender but still have a crisp texture.
4. Stir the veggies and the drained chickpeas together.
5. Combine rice vinegar, hoisin sauce, and soy sauce in a small bowl. After adding the sauce, toss to ensure that the veggies and chickpeas are uniformly coated.

6. Stir-fry the chickpeas for a further two to three minutes, or until they are well cooked.

7. Add sesame seeds to the stir-fry, if using, and toss to mix.

8. Spoon the Chickpea and Vegetable Stir-Fry over warm quinoa or brown rice.

9. You can choose to add sliced green onions as a garnish.

7. Turkey and Avocado Lettuce Wraps

Ingredients:

- 1 lb ground turkey (or cooked turkey breast, shredded)
- 1 avocado, diced
- 1/2 red bell pepper, diced
- 1/4 red onion, finely chopped
- 1/4 cup fresh cilantro, chopped
- Juice of 1 lime
- Salt and pepper to taste
- Lettuce leaves (such as butter lettuce, romaine, or iceberg) for wrapping
- **Optional toppings**: diced tomatoes, shredded cheese, salsa, sour cream

Instructions:

1. In a skillet over medium heat, brown and fully cook the ground turkey, if using. Empty any extra fat. Use your hands or forks to shred the cooked turkey breast.

2. Add the diced avocado, diced red bell pepper, finely sliced red onion, chopped cilantro, and cooked turkey (or shredded turkey breast) to a large mixing bowl.

3. Drizzle with the lime juice and stir everything together.

4. Add salt and pepper to taste when spicing the turkey and avocado combination.

5. Using individual lettuce leaves as wraps, spoon the turkey and avocado mixture onto them.

6. Optional: Top the turkey mixture with extras like sour cream, salsa, shredded cheese, or sliced tomatoes.

7. Using toothpicks if necessary, roll up the lettuce leaves to enclose the filling.

8. Present Turkey and Avocado Lettuce Wraps right away, and savor them as a nutritious and light meal!

8. Eggplant and Tomato Caprese Salad

Ingredients:

- 1 large eggplant, sliced into rounds

- 1-2 large tomatoes, sliced
- Fresh mozzarella cheese, sliced
- Fresh basil leaves
- Balsamic glaze (store-bought or homemade)
- Extra virgin olive oil
- Salt and pepper to taste

Instructions:

1. Turn the heat up to medium-high on your grill or grill pan.
2. Add salt and pepper to the eggplant slices after brushing them with olive oil.
3. Grill the eggplant slices until they are soft and have grill marks, 3 to 4 minutes on each side.
4. Arrange the tomato slices, grilled eggplant pieces, and fresh mozzarella cheese on a serving plate.
5. Insert a few fresh basil leaves between each slice.
6. Drizzle the salad with extra virgin olive oil and balsamic glaze.
7. To taste, add more salt and pepper for seasoning.
8. You can choose to add extra fresh basil leaves as a garnish.

9. Shrimp and Broccoli Quinoa Bowl

Ingredients:

- 1 cup quinoa, rinsed

- 1 lb shrimp, peeled and deveined

- 2 cups broccoli florets

- 2 cloves garlic, minced

- 2 tablespoons olive oil

- 2 tablespoons soy sauce (or tamari for gluten-free option)

- 1 tablespoon honey or maple syrup

- 1 tablespoon rice vinegar

- 1 teaspoon sesame oil

- Salt and pepper to taste

- **Optional garnishes:** sesame seeds, sliced green onions

Instructions:

1. Prepare the quinoa as directed on the box. After cooking, use a fork to fluff and leave aside.

2. To create the sauce, combine the soy sauce, rice vinegar, honey (or maple syrup), and sesame oil in a small bowl. Put aside.

3. In a large pan over medium heat, warm up 1 tablespoon of olive oil. Cook the minced garlic for one to two minutes, or until it becomes aromatic.

4. Put the shrimp in the skillet and cook them for two to three minutes on each side, or until they become opaque and pink. After taking the shrimp out of the pan, set it aside.

5. Place the broccoli florets and the last tablespoon of olive oil in the same skillet. Cook, tossing occasionally, until the broccoli is crisp-tender, about 4–5 minutes.
6. Add the cooked shrimp and broccoli back to the skillet.
7. Cover the shrimp and broccoli in the skillet with the prepared sauce. In order to ensure that everything is equally coated, cook for a further one to two minutes.
8. Distribute the cooked quinoa among bowls for serving. Place the combination of shrimp and broccoli on top.
9. If preferred, garnish with sliced green onions and sesame seeds.
10. Present the Quinoa Bowl with Shrimp and Broccoli right away and savor!

10. Roasted Vegetable and Hummus Wrap

Ingredients:

- 1 large whole-grain or spinach tortilla
- 1 cup mixed roasted vegetables (zucchini, bell peppers, cherry tomatoes, etc.)
- 1/4 cup hummus (store-bought or homemade)

- Handful of fresh spinach leaves
- 1/4 cup feta cheese, crumbled (optional)
- Salt and pepper to taste
- Olive oil for roasting vegetables

Instructions:

1. Set the oven temperature to 400°F, or 200°C.
2. Add salt, pepper, and a sprinkle of olive oil to the mixed veggies. Roast for 20 to 25 minutes, or until soft and beginning to caramelize, in a preheated oven.
3. To make the tortilla more malleable, briefly reheat it in the oven or on a griddle.
4. Evenly cover the tortilla's center with hummus.
5. Top the hummus with the roasted veggies.
6. If wanted, top with crumbled feta cheese and fresh spinach leaves.
7. To make a wrap, fold the tortilla in half along the edges and roll it up from the bottom.
8. You might choose to split the wrap in half to make handling it simpler.

11. Cauliflower Rice and Black Bean Burrito Bowl

Ingredients:

- 1 head cauliflower, riced (or about 4 cups cauliflower rice)
- 1 can (15 oz) black beans, rinsed and drained
- 1 cup corn kernels (fresh, canned, or frozen)
- 1 red bell pepper, diced
- 1/2 red onion, diced
- 2 cloves garlic, minced
- 1 teaspoon ground cumin
- 1 teaspoon chili powder
- Salt and pepper to taste
- 1 tablespoon olive oil
- **Optional toppings:** diced tomatoes, sliced avocado, shredded cheese, chopped cilantro, salsa, lime wedges

Instructions:

1. Rice the cauliflower, if you haven't previously, by chopping it into florets and pounding it in a food processor until it looks like rice. Put aside.

2. In a big skillet over medium heat, warm up the olive oil. Add the minced garlic, red onion, and chopped bell pepper. Simmer for 2 to 3 minutes, or until tender.

3. Add the cauliflower rice to the skillet and toss periodically while cooking for 4–5 minutes, or until the rice begins to soften.

4. Add the corn kernels and black beans and stir. Add chili powder, ground cumin, salt, and pepper for seasoning. Cook everything through for a further two to three minutes.

5. Taste and, if necessary, adjust seasoning.

6. Take the skillet off of the burner once it has fully heated.

7. To serve, portion the black bean mixture and cauliflower rice into individual serving dishes.

8. Garnish with optional toppings like salsa, lime wedges, shredded cheese, diced tomatoes, sliced avocado, and chopped cilantro.

9. Present the Black Bean and Cauliflower Rice Burrito Bowl right away and savor!

12. Mango Salsa Grilled Chicken

Ingredients:

For the Chicken:

- 4 boneless, skinless chicken breasts
- 2 tablespoons olive oil
- 1 teaspoon ground cumin
- 1 teaspoon smoked paprika
- Salt and pepper to taste

For the Mango Salsa:

- 2 ripe mangoes, peeled, pitted, and diced
- 1/2 red onion, finely chopped
- 1 red bell pepper, diced
- 1 jalapeño, seeds removed and finely chopped
- 1/4 cup fresh cilantro, chopped
- Juice of 1 lime
- Salt to taste

Instructions:

1. Turn the heat up to medium-high on the grill.
2. Combine olive oil, smoked paprika, ground cumin, salt, and pepper in a bowl. Distribute this mixture over each chicken breast.
3. Cook the chicken breasts for 6 to 8 minutes on each side, or until they are cooked through and have grill marks. Depending on the thickness of the chicken, cooking times might change.
4. Make the mango salsa while the chicken is grilling. Diced mangos, red onion, red bell pepper, jalapeño, cilantro, lime juice, and salt should all be combined in a dish. Blend well.
5. After the chicken is done, take it off the grill and give it some time to rest.
6. Spoon a heaping tablespoon of mango salsa over each cooked chicken breast.
7. You may pair the Mango Salsa Grilled Chicken with quinoa, rice, or a side salad of your choosing.

13. Quinoa and Spinach Stuffed Portobello Mushrooms

Ingredients:

- 4 large Portobello mushrooms
- 1 cup cooked quinoa
- 2 cups fresh spinach, chopped
- 1/2 cup cherry tomatoes, diced
- 1/4 cup red onion, finely chopped
- 2 cloves garlic, minced
- 1/4 cup grated Parmesan cheese (or nutritional yeast for vegan option)
- 2 tablespoons olive oil
- 1 tablespoon balsamic vinegar
- Salt and pepper to taste
- Fresh parsley or basil for garnish (optional)

Instructions:

1. Turn the oven on to 375°F, or 190°C. Use parchment paper to line a baking sheet.
2. Use a moist paper towel to carefully wipe the Portobello mushrooms. With a spoon, carefully scrape out the gills after removing the stems.

3. Place the cooked quinoa, chopped spinach, sliced cherry tomatoes, finely chopped red onion, minced garlic, nutritional yeast or Parmesan cheese, olive oil, and balsamic vinegar in a large mixing dish. To taste, add salt and pepper for seasoning. To thoroughly mix all components, mix well.

4. Put the Portobello mushrooms, gill side up, on the baking sheet that has been prepared.

5. Tightly compress the quinoa and spinach mixture inside each mushroom, using a little pressure.

6. For extra moisture, drizzle a little olive oil over the packed mushrooms.

7. Bake for 20 to 25 minutes, or until the mixture is cooked through and the mushrooms are soft.

8. When the stuffed Portobello mushrooms are done, take them out of the oven and allow them to cool slightly.

9. If preferred, garnish before serving with fresh basil or parsley.

10. Serve the hot Quinoa and Spinach Stuffed Portobello Mushrooms as a tasty and wholesome side dish or main course for vegetarians.

14. Tofu and Vegetable Skewers with Brown Rice

Ingredients:

For Tofu and Vegetable Skewers:

- 1 block firm tofu, pressed and cubed
- 1 zucchini, sliced into rounds
- 1 red bell pepper, cut into chunks
- 1 red onion, cut into chunks
- Cherry tomatoes
- 2 tablespoons soy sauce
- 1 tablespoon olive oil
- 1 teaspoon garlic powder
- 1 teaspoon smoked paprika
- Salt and pepper to taste
- Wooden skewers, soaked in water

For Brown Rice:

- 1 cup brown rice
- 2 cups water
- Salt to taste

Instructions:

1. Turn the heat up to medium-high on your grill or grill pan.
2. Put the cubed tofu, cherry tomatoes, red bell pepper and red onion pieces, and zucchini rounds in a bowl.

3. Combine the soy sauce, olive oil, smoked paprika, garlic powder, salt, and pepper in another small bowl.

4. Drizzle the tofu and veggies with the marinade, and toss to cover thoroughly. Give it a minimum of 15 to 20 minutes to marinate.

5. Thread the veggies and seasoned tofu onto moistened wooden skewers.

6. Grill the skewers for ten to twelve minutes, rotating them now and again, or until the veggies are soft and the tofu is golden.

7. Make the brown rice while the skewers are roasting. Use cold water to rinse the brown rice. Put the brown rice, water, and a small amount of salt in a pot. After bringing to a boil, lower the heat to a simmer, cover, and cook the rice for 40 to 45 minutes, or until it is tender and the water has been absorbed.

8. Place the vegetable and tofu skewers on top of a bed of brown rice.

15. Greek Salad with Grilled Chicken

Ingredients:

For the Greek Salad:

- 4 boneless, skinless chicken breasts

- 1 tablespoon olive oil
- 1 teaspoon dried oregano
- Salt and pepper to taste
- 4 cups mixed salad greens (such as lettuce, spinach, arugula)
- 1 cucumber, sliced
- 1 cup cherry tomatoes, halved
- 1/2 red onion, thinly sliced
- 1/2 cup Kalamata olives, pitted
- 1/2 cup crumbled feta cheese
- Fresh parsley or oregano for garnish (optional)

For the Greek Salad Dressing:

- 1/4 cup extra virgin olive oil
- 2 tablespoons red wine vinegar
- 1 clove garlic, minced
- 1 teaspoon dried oregano
- Salt and pepper to taste

Instructions:

For the Grilled Chicken:

1. Turn the heat up to medium-high on the grill.
2. Combine the olive oil, salt, pepper, and dried oregano in a small dish.
3. Apply the olive oil mixture to both sides of the chicken breasts.

4. Grill the chicken breasts for 6 to 8 minutes on each side, or until they are well cooked and the middle is no longer pink. A temperature of 165°F (75°C) should be reached inside.

5. After the chicken is done, take it from the grill and give it some time to rest before slicing.

For the Greek Salad:

1. Combine the mixed salad greens, cucumber slices, cherry tomatoes, red onion slices that have been thinly cut, crumbled feta cheese, and Kalamata olives in a large mixing bowl.

2. Combine the extra virgin olive oil, red wine vinegar, minced garlic, dried oregano, salt, and pepper in a small bowl to make the Greek Salad Dressing.

3. Drizzle the salad ingredients in the mixing basin with the dressing, tossing to evenly coat.

To Serve:

1. Distribute the Greek salad among plates for serving.

2. After grilling, cut the chicken breasts into slices and place them over the salad.

3. If preferred, garnish with fresh oregano or parsley.

4. Present the Greek salad with grilled chicken right away, then savor it!

16. *Sweet Potato and Kale Hash*

Ingredients:

- 2 medium sweet potatoes, peeled and diced
- 1 bunch kale, stems removed and leaves chopped
- 1 onion, finely chopped
- 2 cloves garlic, minced
- 2 tablespoons olive oil
- 1 teaspoon smoked paprika
- 1/2 teaspoon cumin
- Salt and pepper to taste
- **Optional toppings:** fried or poached eggs, avocado slices, hot sauce

Instructions:

1. Heat the olive oil in a big pan over medium-high heat.
2. Include chopped onion and cook for two to three minutes, or until tender.
3. Fill the pan with chopped sweet potatoes. Sweet potatoes should be cooked for 8 to 10 minutes, stirring now and again, until they are soft and golden.

4. Add the minced garlic to the skillet and cook it for one to two more minutes, or until it becomes aromatic.

5. Add the cumin, smoked paprika, chopped kale, salt, and pepper. Cook the kale for three to five minutes, or until it's soft and wilted.

6. If necessary, taste and adjust the spices.

7. You can add more protein to the Sweet Potato and Kale Hash by serving it with fried or poached eggs on top.

8. If preferred, garnish with slices of avocado and a splash of spicy sauce.

17. Turkey and Vegetable Quiche

Ingredients:

- 1 prepared pie crust (store-bought or homemade)
- 1 tablespoon olive oil
- 1/2 lb ground turkey
- 1 small onion, diced
- 1 bell pepper, diced
- 1 cup chopped spinach or kale
- 1/2 cup cherry tomatoes, halved
- 6 large eggs
- 1/2 cup milk (dairy or plant-based)
- 1/2 cup shredded cheese (such as cheddar, mozzarella, or Swiss)

- Salt and pepper to taste
- **Optional**: herbs or spices of your choice (such as dried thyme, basil, or smoked paprika)

Instructions:

1. Set the oven temperature to 375°F, or 190°C.
2. Press the prepared pie dough into a 9-inch pie plate after rolling it out. Cut off any extra crust that is hanging over the sides.
3. Heat the olive oil in a pan over medium heat. Cook the bell pepper and chopped onion for approximately five minutes, or until they are tender.
4. Add the ground turkey to the skillet and heat, breaking it up with a spoon, until it is browned and cooked through.
5. Add the chopped kale or spinach and simmer for 2 minutes, or until wilted. Take off the heat and let it cool a little.
6. Stir the eggs and milk together thoroughly in a mixing basin. Add salt, pepper, and any other desired herbs or spices for seasoning.
7. Evenly cover the bottom of the prepared pie crust with the cooked turkey and vegetable mixture. Add a few cherry tomatoes on top.
8. Cover the veggies and turkey in the pie shell with the egg mixture.
9. Top the quiche with cheese that has been shredded.

10. After preheating the oven, put the quiche in and bake it for thirty to thirty-five minutes, or until the top is golden brown and the middle is set.

11. After the quiche is done, take it out of the oven and allow it to cool down before cutting into slices and serving.

18. Whole Wheat Pita Bread with Hummus and Veggies

Ingredients:

- 4 whole wheat pita bread rounds
- 1 cup hummus (store-bought or homemade)
- 1 cucumber, thinly sliced
- 1 bell pepper, thinly sliced
- 1 carrot, grated or thinly sliced
- 1/4 red onion, thinly sliced
- Handful of cherry tomatoes, halved
- Handful of mixed salad greens
- **Optional toppings:** olives, feta cheese, avocado slices, sprouts

Instructions:

1. Heat the whole wheat pita bread rounds on a hot skillet or in a toaster oven until they are lightly crispy and thoroughly toasted.

2. On each round of hot pita bread, spread a thick layer of hummus.

3. Arrange the bell pepper, carrot, cherry tomatoes, red onion, cucumber slices, and mixed salad greens on top of the hummus.

4. Top with any optional ingredients you like, such sprouts, avocado slices, feta cheese, or olives.

5. The pita bread can be rolled up like a wrap or folded in half.

6. Present the Whole Wheat Pita Bread along with the Hummus and vegetables right away, and savor!

19. Zucchini Noodles with Pesto and Cherry Tomatoes

Ingredients:

- 4 medium-sized zucchini, spiralized into noodles
- 1 cup cherry tomatoes, halved
- 1/2 cup fresh basil leaves
- 1/3 cup pine nuts, toasted
- 1/2 cup grated Parmesan cheese
- 2 cloves garlic, minced
- 1/2 cup extra virgin olive oil

- Salt and pepper to taste
- **Optional:** Red pepper flakes for a hint of spice

Instructions:

1. Put the fresh basil, roasted pine nuts, grated Parmesan cheese, chopped garlic, and a dash of salt in a food processor. Blend the items until they are well-chopped.
2. Add the olive oil little by little while the food processor is running, until the pesto has a smooth consistency. To taste, add salt and pepper for seasoning.
3. Heat a little amount of olive oil in a big skillet over medium heat. Sauté the zucchini noodles for two to three minutes, or until they are somewhat soft.
4. Cook the cherry tomatoes in the pan for a further one to two minutes, or until they begin to soften.
5. Gently toss the cherry tomatoes and zucchini noodles in the prepared pesto until well covered.
6. For a little kick of heat, feel free to top with red pepper flakes.
7. Present the Pesto and Cherry Tomatoes over Zucchini Noodles right away.

20. Spinach and Feta Stuffed Chicken Breast

Ingredients:

- 4 boneless, skinless chicken breasts
- 2 cups fresh spinach leaves
- 1/2 cup crumbled feta cheese
- 2 cloves garlic, minced
- 1 tablespoon olive oil
- 1 teaspoon dried oregano
- Salt and pepper to taste
- Toothpicks or kitchen twine

Instructions:

1. Set the oven temperature to 375°F, or 190°C.
2. Heat the olive oil in a skillet over medium heat. When aromatic, add the minced garlic and simmer for one to two minutes.
3. Cook the fresh spinach leaves in the pan for two to three minutes, or until they have wilted. Take off the heat and let it cool a little.
4. After the cooked spinach has cooled, wring out any extra liquid.
5. Add the crumbled feta cheese to a mixing dish along with the wilted spinach. Add salt, pepper, and dried oregano to the dish and stir well.

6. To create a pocket for the filling, score each chicken breast horizontally with a sharp knife. Take cautious not to slice through completely.

7. Divide the spinach and feta mixture equally among the chicken breasts and stuff each one.

8. To keep the filling from spilling out, fasten the chicken breast holes with toothpicks or kitchen twine.

9. Sprinkle some dried oregano and salt and pepper on the exterior of the chicken breasts.

10. Transfer the packed chicken breasts to a baking dish that has been gently oiled or covered with parchment paper.

11. Bake for 25 to 30 minutes, or until the chicken is cooked through and the internal temperature reaches 165°F (75°C), in the preheated oven.

12. When the chicken breasts are done, take them out of the oven and give them a few minutes to rest before serving.

13. If wanted, top the hot spinach and feta stuffed chicken breast with fresh herbs.

CHAPTER FIVE: DELICIOUS AND MOUTHWATERING DINNERS

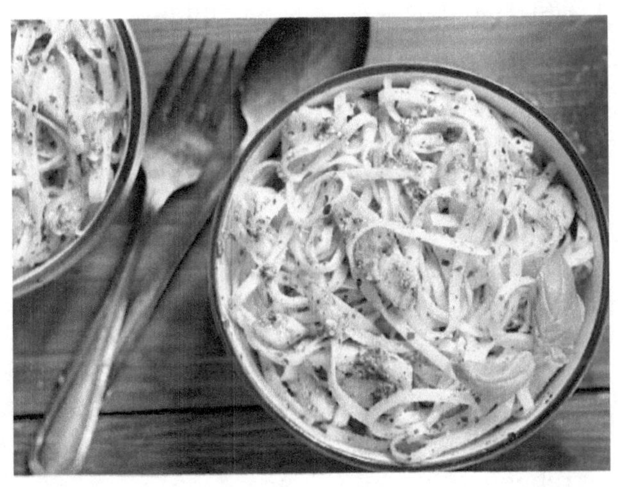

1. Grilled Salmon with Lemon-Dill Sauce

Ingredients:

- 4 salmon filets
- 2 tablespoons olive oil
- Salt and pepper to taste
- Lemon wedges for serving

For the Lemon-Dill Sauce:

- 1/2 cup Greek yogurt
- 2 tablespoons fresh lemon juice
- 1 tablespoon chopped fresh dill (or 1 teaspoon dried dill)
- 1 clove garlic, minced
- Salt and pepper to taste

Instructions:

For the Grilled Salmon:

1. Turn the heat up to medium-high on your grill.
2. Season the salmon filets with salt and pepper after rubbing olive oil on both sides.
3. Skin-side down, put the salmon filets on the hot grill.
4. Cook the salmon on the grill for 4–5 minutes on each side, or until it is cooked through and flake readily with a fork.

5. After the salmon is done, take it off the grill and place it on a dish for serving.

6. Present the hot salmon that has been cooked, accompanied by lemon wedges.

For the Lemon-Dill Sauce:

1. Combine Greek yogurt, minced garlic, chopped dill, fresh lemon juice, salt, and pepper in a small bowl. Mix well until creamy and smooth.

2. If necessary, taste and adjust the seasoning.

3. Present the grilled salmon with the Lemon-Dill Sauce on the side.

2. Mediterranean Chickpea Salad Bowl

Ingredients:

For the Salad:

- 2 cups cooked chickpeas (or 1 can, rinsed and drained)
- 1 cucumber, diced
- 1 bell pepper (red, yellow, or orange), diced
- 1 cup cherry tomatoes, halved
- 1/4 red onion, thinly sliced

- 1/2 cup pitted Kalamata olives, halved
- 1/4 cup crumbled feta cheese (optional)
- Handful of fresh parsley, chopped
- Handful of fresh mint leaves, chopped (optional)

For the Dressing:

- 1/4 cup extra virgin olive oil
- 2 tablespoons freshly squeezed lemon juice
- 1 clove garlic, minced
- 1 teaspoon dried oregano
- Salt and pepper to taste

Optional Extras:

- Cooked quinoa or couscous
- Sliced avocado
- Grilled chicken or tofu

Instructions:

1. The cooked chickpeas, diced cucumber, diced bell pepper, split cherry tomatoes, thinly sliced red onion, halved Kalamata olives, crumbled feta cheese (if using), chopped parsley, and chopped mint leaves (if used) should all be combined in a large mixing dish.

2. Combine the extra virgin olive oil, lemon juice, minced garlic, dried oregano, salt, and pepper in a small bowl to make the dressing.

3. Drizzle the ingredients for the chickpea salad in the mixing bowl with the dressing. Toss to ensure that the dressing coats everything equally.

4. Taste and, if necessary, adjust seasoning.

5. You can choose to serve the Mediterranean Chickpea Salad with grilled chicken or tofu on top, cooked quinoa or couscous, or sliced avocado as optional toppings.

6. You may either serve the salad right away or save it for later. It can be served at room temperature or cold.

3. Vegetable and Quinoa Stuffed Bell Peppers

Ingredients:

- 4 large bell peppers, any color
- 1 cup quinoa, rinsed
- 2 cups vegetable broth or water
- 1 tablespoon olive oil
- 1 small onion, diced
- 2 cloves garlic, minced
- 1 carrot, diced

- 1 zucchini, diced
- 1 cup cherry tomatoes, halved
- 1 cup cooked black beans (or canned, rinsed and drained)
- 1 teaspoon ground cumin
- 1 teaspoon smoked paprika
- Salt and pepper to taste
- 1/4 cup chopped fresh parsley or cilantro
- 1/2 cup shredded cheese (such as cheddar, mozzarella, or pepper jack), optional

Instructions:

1. Set the oven temperature to 375°F, or 190°C.
2. Slice off the bell peppers' tops, then take out the seeds and membranes. Put aside.
3. Place the quinoa and water or vegetable broth in a medium pot. After bringing to a boil, lower the heat to a simmer, cover, and cook the quinoa for 15 to 20 minutes, or until it is tender and the liquid has been absorbed.
4. Heat the olive oil in a big pan over medium heat. Add the chopped onion and garlic, and simmer for 3–4 minutes, or until softened.
5. Cook the chopped zucchini and carrot in the pan for a further four to five minutes, or until the veggies are soft.

6. Add the cooked black beans and cherry tomatoes cut in half and cook for 2 to 3 minutes, or until well cooked.

7. Add salt, pepper, smoked paprika, and ground cumin to the vegetable mixture and toss to incorporate.

8. Include the cooked quinoa in the skillet along with the veggies, and thoroughly stir to include all the ingredients. Take off the heat.

9. Add finely chopped cilantro or parsley.

10. Add half of the shredded cheese, if using, to the quinoa and veggie combination.

11. Evenly distribute the quinoa and veggie mixture among the hollowed-out bell peppers using a spoon.

12. With the bell peppers packed, place them upright in a baking dish.

13. **Optional:** Top the filled bell peppers with the leftover shredded cheese.

14. Bake the baking dish for 25 to 30 minutes in a preheated oven covered with aluminum foil.

15. Take off the foil and continue baking for a further five to ten minutes, or until the cheese is bubbling and melted and the bell peppers are soft.

16. Before serving, take the cooked filled bell peppers out of the oven and allow them to cool for a few minutes.

4. Baked Cod with Herbed Quinoa

Ingredients:

For the Baked Cod:

- 4 cod filets (about 6 oz each)
- 2 tablespoons olive oil
- Salt and pepper to taste
- 2 cloves garlic, minced
- 1 lemon, sliced
- 1 tablespoon chopped fresh herbs (such as parsley, dill, or thyme)
- Lemon wedges for serving

For the Herbed Quinoa:

- 1 cup quinoa, rinsed
- 2 cups vegetable broth or water
- 2 tablespoons chopped fresh herbs (such as parsley, dill, or chives)
- 2 tablespoons freshly squeezed lemon juice
- Salt and pepper to taste

Instructions:

For the Baked Cod:

1. Set the oven temperature to 375°F, or 190°C.

2. Using paper towels, pat the cod filets dry before putting them on a baking dish.
3. Season the cod filets to taste with salt and pepper and drizzle with olive oil.
4. Sprinkle the filets with chopped fresh herbs and top each one with a few lemon slices after rubbing the filets with minced garlic.
5. Bake the cod for 15 to 20 minutes, or until it is cooked through and flakes readily with a fork, in the preheated oven.
6. After the cod is done, take it out of the oven and give it a few minutes to rest before serving.

For the Herbed Quinoa:

1. Place the quinoa and water or vegetable broth in a medium pot. After bringing to a boil, lower the heat to a simmer, cover, and cook the quinoa for 15 to 20 minutes, or until it is tender and the liquid has been absorbed.
2. Using a fork, fluff the cooked quinoa and mix in the freshly squeezed lemon juice, chopped fresh herbs, salt, and pepper to taste.

To Serve:

1. Distribute the quinoa with herbs among serving dishes.

2. Top each serving of quinoa with a baked cod filet.

3. If wanted, garnish with more lemon wedges and fresh herbs.

4. Present the baked cod with herb quinoa right away, then savor it!

5. *Teriyaki Turkey Stir-Fry*

Ingredients:

- 1 lb turkey breast or turkey tenderloin, thinly sliced
- 2 tablespoons soy sauce (or tamari for gluten-free option)
- 2 tablespoons teriyaki sauce
- 1 tablespoon rice vinegar
- 1 tablespoon honey or maple syrup
- 2 cloves garlic, minced
- 1 tablespoon sesame oil
- 1 tablespoon vegetable oil
- 1 onion, thinly sliced
- 1 bell pepper, thinly sliced
- 1 cup broccoli florets
- 1 carrot, julienned
- 1 cup snow peas, trimmed
- Cooked rice or noodles for serving

- Sesame seeds and sliced green onions for garnish (optional)

Instructions:

1. To create the teriyaki marinade, combine the soy sauce, teriyaki sauce, rice vinegar, honey or maple syrup, and chopped garlic in a small bowl.

2. Transfer the thinly sliced turkey to a sealable plastic bag or a shallow plate. Transfer half of the teriyaki marinade onto the turkey; save aside remaining marinade for later use. Toss the turkey in the marinade to ensure uniform coating. Let it marinade for a minimum of half an hour and a maximum of two hours in the fridge.

3. In a large skillet or wok, heat the vegetable and sesame oils over medium-high heat.

4. Add the turkey slices that have marinated, being sure to remove any extra marinade. The turkey should be cooked through and browned after two to three minutes on each side. After taking the turkey out of the skillet, set it aside.

5. Add the bell pepper, broccoli florets, julienned carrot, sliced onion, and snow peas to the same skillet. When the veggies are crisp-tender, stir-fry them for four to five minutes.

6. Add the cooked turkey and veggies back to the skillet.

7. Cover the turkey and veggies in the skillet with the leftover teriyaki marinade. In order to uniformly cover everything with sauce, stir.

8. Cook for a further one to two minutes, or until the turkey and veggies are coated in a little thicker sauce.

9. Over cooked rice or noodles, serve the hot Teriyaki Turkey Stir-Fry.

10. If preferred, garnish with sliced green onions and sesame seeds.

6. *Spaghetti Squash with Tomato Basil Sauce*

Ingredients:

- 1 medium spaghetti squash
- 2 tablespoons olive oil
- Salt and pepper to taste
- 2 cloves garlic, minced
- 1 can (14 oz) crushed tomatoes
- 1/4 cup chopped fresh basil
- 1 teaspoon dried oregano
- 1/2 teaspoon red pepper flakes (optional)
- Grated Parmesan cheese for serving (optional)

Instructions:

Set the oven temperature to 400°F, or 200°C.

2. Scoop out the seeds and fibrous strands with a spoon after cutting the spaghetti squash in half lengthwise.

3. Season with salt and pepper and drizzle olive oil over the sliced sides of the spaghetti squash halves.

4. Lay the spaghetti squash halves on a baking sheet covered with parchment paper, cut side down.

5. Roast the spaghetti squash for 35 to 45 minutes, or until a fork can easily penetrate it into the flesh.

6. Make the tomato-basil sauce while the spaghetti squash roasts. In a saucepan, warm the olive oil over medium heat.

7. Cook the minced garlic in the saucepan for one to two minutes, or until it becomes aromatic.

8. Add the red pepper flakes (if using), chopped fresh basil, dry oregano, and smashed tomatoes. To taste, add salt and pepper for seasoning.

9. To let the flavors melt together, simmer the sauce for ten to fifteen minutes, stirring now and again.

10. After the spaghetti squash is soft and roasted, scrape the flesh into strands with a fork to make "spaghetti."

11. Spoon spaghetti squash strands onto serving dishes, then drizzle with tomato basil sauce.

12. **Optional:** Before serving, top with grated Parmesan cheese.

13. Enjoy your delicious spaghetti squash with tomato basil sauce!

7. *Cauliflower Crust Margherita Pizza*

Ingredients:

For the Cauliflower Crust:

- 1 medium-sized cauliflower, riced (about 4 cups)
- 1/2 cup shredded mozzarella cheese
- 1/4 cup grated Parmesan cheese
- 1/2 teaspoon dried oregano
- 1/2 teaspoon garlic powder
- 2 large eggs
- Salt and pepper to taste

For Toppings:

- 1/2 cup pizza sauce
- 1 1/2 cups fresh mozzarella cheese, sliced
- 2-3 ripe tomatoes, sliced
- Fresh basil leaves
- Olive oil for drizzling (optional)
- Salt and pepper to taste

Instructions:

1. Set the oven's temperature to 425°F (220°C). As the oven heats up, place a baking sheet or pizza stone inside.
2. Use a box grater or food processor to rice the cauliflower. After ricing, place the cauliflower in a clean kitchen towel and wring off any extra liquid.
3. Combine the riced cauliflower, eggs, salt, pepper, dried oregano, grated Parmesan, shredded mozzarella, and garlic powder in a bowl. Blend until well blended.
4. Line another baking sheet or a pizza peel with parchment paper. Forming the cauliflower mixture into a circular pizza crust, spread it out onto the parchment paper.
5. Gently place the parchment paper containing the crust onto the baking sheet or pizza stone that has been warmed.
6. Bake for 15 to 20 minutes, or until the cauliflower crust is crisp and golden.
7. Take the crust out of the oven and cover it with pizza sauce. Place tomatoes and sliced fresh mozzarella over top.
8. Put the pizza back in the oven and bake it for ten to twelve more minutes, or until the cheese is bubbling and melted.
9. Add some fresh basil leaves to the Cauliflower Crust Margherita Pizza once it comes out of the

oven. If preferred, drizzle with olive oil and add salt and pepper for seasoning.

10. Cut into slices and savor your low-carb margherita pizza with cauliflower crust!

8. Lemon Garlic Shrimp Skewers with Brown Rice

Ingredients:

For the Shrimp Skewers:

- 1 lb large shrimp, peeled and deveined
- Zest and juice of 1 lemon
- 3 cloves garlic, minced
- 2 tablespoons olive oil
- Salt and pepper to taste
- Wooden or metal skewers

For the Brown Rice:

- 1 cup brown rice
- 2 cups water or vegetable broth
- Salt to taste

Optional Garnish:

- Chopped fresh parsley
- Lemon wedges

Instructions:

For the Shrimp Skewers:

1. To avoid burning, soak wooden skewers in water for at least half an hour before using them.
2. Add the olive oil, minced garlic, lemon zest, lemon juice, salt, and pepper to a mixing bowl.
3. Transfer the peeled and deveined shrimp to the bowl and mix to ensure that the marinade coats them evenly. In the fridge, let the shrimp marinade for at least 15 to 30 minutes.
4. Distribute the marinated shrimp evenly among the skewers by threading them onto them.
5. Turn the heat up to medium-high on your grill or grill pan.
6. Grill the shrimp skewers until they are opaque and pink, about two to three minutes each side.
7. After the shrimp skewers are done, take them off the grill and lay them aside.

For the Brown Rice:

1. Put the brown rice and the vegetable broth or water in a pot. To taste, add salt.

2. Once the mixture reaches a boil, lower the heat to a simmer, cover, and let the rice cook for 40 to 45 minutes, or until it is soft and the liquid has been absorbed.
3. Using a fork, fluff the cooked brown rice.

To Serve:

1. Transfer cooked brown rice onto each serving plate.
2. Top the brown rice with the grilled lemon garlic shrimp skewers.
3. Optional: For added taste, garnish with lemon wedges and finely chopped fresh parsley.
4. Present the heated Lemon Garlic Shrimp Skewers beside Brown Rice and savor!

9. Stuffed Zucchini Boats with Ground Turkey

Ingredients:

- 4 medium zucchini
- 1 lb ground turkey
- 1 onion, finely chopped
- 2 cloves garlic, minced
- 1 bell pepper, diced

- 1 cup cherry tomatoes, halved
- 1 teaspoon dried oregano
- 1 teaspoon dried basil
- Salt and pepper to taste
- 1 cup shredded mozzarella cheese
- Fresh parsley for garnish (optional)
- Olive oil for cooking

Instructions:

1. Set the oven temperature to 375°F, or 190°C.
2. To produce boat-shaped halves, cut the zucchini in half lengthwise and use a spoon to scoop out the centers. Keep the zucchini that you scooped out for later.
3. Heat the olive oil in a big pan over medium heat. Add the chopped onion and garlic, and cook until they become soft.
4. Add the ground turkey to the skillet and heat, breaking it up with a spoon as it cooks, until it is browned.
5. Chop the zucchini that was set aside in step 2 and combine it with the diced bell pepper, cherry tomatoes, dried basil, dried oregano, and salt and pepper in the pan. Cook the veggies for a further five to seven minutes, or until they are soft.
6. Spoon the ground turkey and vegetable mixture into each zucchini boat.

7. Cover the top of each filled zucchini boat with shredded mozzarella.

8. Put the packed boats made of zucchini into a baking dish.

9. Bake for 20 to 25 minutes in a preheated oven, or until the zucchini is soft and the cheese is bubbling.

10. Before serving, you can optionally garnish with fresh parsley.

10. Mushroom and Spinach Frittata

Ingredients:

- 8 large eggs
- 1 cup mushrooms, sliced
- 2 cups fresh spinach, chopped
- 1/2 onion, finely chopped
- 2 cloves garlic, minced
- 1/2 cup shredded mozzarella cheese
- 1/4 cup grated Parmesan cheese
- 2 tablespoons olive oil
- Salt and pepper to taste
- Fresh herbs (such as parsley or chives) for garnish (optional)

Instructions:

1. Set the oven temperature to 175°C, or 350°F.

2. Heat the olive oil in a large oven-safe pan over medium heat.

3. Include the diced onion and sauté until it becomes soft. Next, include the sliced mushrooms and cook them until they release their moisture and turn golden brown.

4. Add the minced garlic to the skillet and cook it for one to two more minutes, or until it becomes aromatic.

5. Cook the chopped spinach in the pan until it wilts.

6. Combine the eggs, Parmesan, mozzarella, and salt and pepper in a bowl.

7. Evenly cover the veggies in the pan with the egg mixture. Give the edges a few minutes to set.

8. Place the pan in the oven that has been warmed, and bake for 15 to 20 minutes, or until the frittata is set through.

9. After cooking, take it out of the oven and give it some time to cool.

10. Before serving, you can choose to garnish with fresh herbs.

11. Grilled Chicken with Mango Avocado Salsa

Ingredients:

For the Grilled Chicken:

- 4 boneless, skinless chicken breasts
- 2 tablespoons olive oil
- 1 teaspoon ground cumin
- 1 teaspoon smoked paprika
- Salt and pepper to taste

For the Mango Avocado Salsa:

- 1 ripe mango, peeled, pitted, and diced
- 1 ripe avocado, peeled, pitted, and diced
- 1/4 cup red onion, finely chopped
- 1/4 cup fresh cilantro, chopped
- Juice of 1 lime
- Salt and pepper to taste

Optional Garnish:

- Sliced jalapeño for a spicy kick
- Chopped fresh cilantro
- Lime wedges

Instructions:

For the Grilled Chicken:

1. Turn the heat up to medium-high on your grill.

2. Combine the olive oil, smoked paprika, ground cumin, salt, and pepper in a small bowl.

3. Apply the olive oil mixture to the chicken breasts on both sides.

4. After preheating the grill, place the chicken breasts on it and cook for 6 to 8 minutes on each side, or until the chicken is cooked through and the middle is no longer pink. A temperature of 165°F (75°C) should be reached inside.

5. After they are done, take the chicken breasts from the grill and give them a few minutes to rest before slicing.

For the Mango Avocado Salsa:

1. Place the diced mango, diced avocado, finely sliced red onion, chopped cilantro, and lime juice in a medium-sized mixing bowl.

2. When making the salsa, add salt and pepper to taste. Gently stir all ingredients together.

To Serve:

1. Transfer the grilled chicken breasts to a serving platter after slicing.

2. Arrange the grilled chicken on top of the Mango Avocado Salsa.

3. **Optional garnish:** For a spicy kick, add slices of jalapeño, lime wedges, and freshly chopped cilantro.

4. Serve the Mango Avocado Salsa alongside the Grilled Chicken immediately and enjoy!

12. *Sweet Potato and Black Bean Enchiladas*

Ingredients:

For the Enchiladas:

- 2 large sweet potatoes, peeled and diced
- 1 tablespoon olive oil
- 1 teaspoon ground cumin
- 1 teaspoon chili powder
- Salt and pepper to taste
- 1 can (15 oz) black beans, drained and rinsed
- 1 cup corn kernels (fresh, frozen, or canned)
- 1/2 cup diced red onion
- 2 cloves garlic, minced
- 1 cup shredded cheese (such as cheddar or Monterey Jack)
- 8-10 large flour tortillas or corn tortillas

For the Enchilada Sauce:

- 2 tablespoons olive oil
- 2 tablespoons all-purpose flour (or gluten-free flour)
- 2 tablespoons chili powder
- 1 teaspoon ground cumin
- 1 teaspoon garlic powder
- 1/2 teaspoon dried oregano
- 2 cups vegetable broth
- 1 can (8 oz) tomato sauce
- Salt and pepper to taste

Optional Garnish:

- Chopped fresh cilantro
- Sliced jalapeños
- Sour cream or Greek yogurt
- Avocado slices
- Lime wedges

Instructions:

For the Enchiladas:

1. Set the oven temperature to 375°F, or 190°C.
2. Heat the olive oil in a big skillet over medium heat. Add the chopped sweet potatoes and season with chili powder, salt, pepper, and ground cumin.

Cook, stirring occasionally, until the sweet potatoes are soft, 10 to 12 minutes.

3. Combine the cooked sweet potatoes, black beans, corn kernels, chopped red onion, and minced garlic in a pan. Cook, stirring, for a further two to three minutes, or until well heated.

4. Turn off the heat source and place the skillet aside.

5. Use a skillet or microwave to reheat the tortillas until they are soft.

6. Evenly distribute the sweet potato and black bean mixture among the tortillas by spooning it onto each one. Top the filling with cheese that has been shredded.

7. Tightly roll up the tortillas, then put them on a baking tray seam-side down.

8. Continue until all of the filling and tortillas have been used.

For the Enchilada Sauce:

1. Heat the olive oil in a saucepan over medium heat. To form a roux, add the all-purpose flour and simmer, stirring frequently, for one to two minutes.

2. After approximately a minute, stir in the dried oregano, powdered cumin, garlic powder, and chili powder until fragrant.

3. Add tomato sauce and vegetable broth gradually, whisking until smooth.

4. Simmer the sauce for five to seven minutes, stirring now and again, until it thickens a little. To taste, add salt and pepper for seasoning.

Assembly and Baking:

After rolling the tortillas, place them in the baking dish and equally cover with the enchilada sauce.
2. You may top with more shredded cheese if you like.
3. Place aluminum foil over the baking dish and bake in the preheated oven for 20 to 25 minutes, or until the cheese is bubbling and melted and the enchiladas are well warm.
4. After cooking, take off the foil and continue baking for a further five minutes, or until the cheese is crisp and golden.
5. Before serving, take the enchiladas out of the oven and let them cool for a few minutes.

To Serve:

1. If preferred, garnish the Sweet Potato and Black Bean Enchiladas with avocado slices, sour cream or Greek yogurt, chopped fresh cilantro, and lime wedges.
2. Present this aromatic and filling meal while it's still hot!

13. Turkey and Vegetable Kabobs with Quinoa

Ingredients:

For Turkey and Vegetable Kabobs:

- 1 lb ground turkey
- 1 zucchini, sliced into rounds
- 1 bell pepper, cut into chunks
- 1 red onion, cut into chunks
- Cherry tomatoes
- 2 tablespoons olive oil
- 1 teaspoon ground cumin
- 1 teaspoon smoked paprika
- Salt and pepper to taste
- Wooden or metal skewers

For Quinoa:

- 1 cup quinoa, rinsed
- 2 cups water or vegetable broth
- Salt to taste

Instructions:

1. Turn the heat up to medium-high on your grill or grill pan.

2. Combine the ground turkey, smoked paprika, olive oil, ground cumin, salt, and pepper in a bowl. Blend well.

3. Thread the seasoned ground turkey onto skewers, alternating with zucchini rounds, bell pepper pieces, red onion chunks, and cherry tomatoes.

4. Grill the kabobs for ten to twelve minutes, rotating them now and again, until the veggies are starting to become a little browned and the turkey is cooked through.

5. Make the quinoa while the kabobs are roasting. Quinoa, water or veggie broth, and a small amount of salt should all be combined in a pot. After bringing to a boil, lower the heat to a simmer, cover, and cook the quinoa for approximately fifteen minutes, or until the water has been absorbed.

6. Spoon the cooked quinoa on top of the turkey and vegetable kabobs.

7. You may either pour some fresh lemon juice or sprinkle some more olive oil on top for taste.

14. Caprese Quinoa Bowl

Ingredients:

- 1 cup quinoa, rinsed
- 2 cups water or vegetable broth
- 2 cups cherry tomatoes, halved
- 1 cup fresh mozzarella balls (bocconcini), halved
- 1/4 cup fresh basil leaves, chopped
- 2 tablespoons extra virgin olive oil
- 1 tablespoon balsamic vinegar
- Salt and pepper to taste
- Balsamic glaze for drizzling (optional)

Instructions:

1. Put the quinoa and the vegetable broth or water in a saucepan. After bringing to a boil, lower the heat to a simmer, cover, and cook the quinoa for 15 to 20 minutes, or until it is tender and the liquid has been absorbed. Using a fork, fluff the quinoa and let it cool somewhat.

2. Place the cooked quinoa, chopped fresh basil leaves, half cherry tomatoes, and halved fresh mozzarella balls in a large mixing bowl.

3. To create the dressing, combine the extra virgin olive oil and balsamic vinegar in a small bowl.

4. Drizzle the quinoa mixture with the dressing, tossing to cover everything thoroughly.

5. Use salt and pepper to taste while preparing the Caprese quinoa bowl.

6. Distribute the combination of quinoa among serving dishes.

7. Optional: For added taste, drizzle balsamic glaze over the top of each bowl.

8. Present the Caprese Quinoa Bowls right away and savor them!

15. Eggplant Parmesan with Whole Wheat Pasta

Ingredients:

For Eggplant Parmesan:

- 2 large eggplants, sliced into rounds
- 2 cups whole wheat breadcrumbs
- 1 cup grated Parmesan cheese
- 2 cups marinara sauce
- 2 cups shredded mozzarella cheese
- 2 tablespoons fresh basil, chopped
- 2 tablespoons olive oil
- Salt and pepper to taste

For Whole Wheat Pasta:

- 2 cups whole wheat pasta
- Salt for boiling

Instructions:

For Eggplant Parmesan:

1. Set the oven temperature to 375°F, or 190°C.
2. Combine whole wheat breadcrumbs, salt, pepper, and grated Parmesan cheese in a bowl.
3. Coat both sides of each eggplant slice by dipping it into the breadcrumb mixture.
4. Place a large pan over medium-high heat with olive oil. Slices of breaded eggplant should be added and cooked for two to three minutes on each side, or until golden brown.
5. Apply a thin layer of marinara sauce to a baking dish. Arrange the browned eggplant slices in a stack on top.
6. Drizzle the eggplant slices with more marinara sauce and top with mozzarella cheese shreds.
7. Continue layering eggplant slices until all of them are utilized, and then top with a layer of mozzarella cheese.
8. Bake for 25 to 30 minutes, or until the cheese is bubbling and melted, in a preheated oven.
9. Before serving, garnish with freshly chopped basil.

For Whole Wheat Pasta:

1. Bring a big saucepan of water that has been salted to a boil.

2. Cook the whole wheat pasta until al dente, following the directions on the package.
3. To avoid sticking, drain the pasta and mix it with a little olive oil.

16. Baked Chicken Breast with Roasted Vegetables

Ingredients:

For Baked Chicken Breast:

- 4 boneless, skinless chicken breasts
- 2 tablespoons olive oil
- 1 teaspoon garlic powder
- 1 teaspoon paprika
- 1 teaspoon dried thyme
- Salt and pepper to taste
- Lemon wedges for serving

For Roasted Vegetables:

- 2 cups baby potatoes, halved
- 2 cups carrots, peeled and sliced
- 2 cups broccoli florets
- 1 red bell pepper, cut into chunks
- 2 tablespoons olive oil

- 1 teaspoon dried rosemary
- Salt and pepper to taste

Instructions:

1. Set the oven's temperature to 425°F (220°C).
2. Combine olive oil, salt, pepper, dried thyme, paprika, and garlic powder in a basin. Apply this mix onto every chicken breast.
3. Transfer the breasts of chicken to a baking dish.
4. Combine olive oil, dried rosemary, salt, and pepper in a separate bowl and toss with small potatoes, carrots, broccoli florets, and red bell pepper.
5. In the baking dish, arrange the seasoned veggies around the chicken breasts.
6. Bake, turning occasionally, in a preheated oven for 25 to 30 minutes, or until the chicken is cooked through and the veggies are soft.
7. **Optional**: To brown the tops of the chicken breasts, broil for a further two to three minutes.
8. Present the Roasted Vegetables with Baked Chicken Breast, accompanied by lemon wedges.

17. Lentil and Vegetable Curry

Ingredients:

- 1 cup dried lentils (green or brown), rinsed and drained
- 2 tablespoons olive oil
- 1 onion, diced
- 3 cloves garlic, minced
- 1 tablespoon fresh ginger, grated
- 2 carrots, diced
- 1 bell pepper, diced
- 1 zucchini, diced
- 1 can (14 oz) diced tomatoes
- 1 can (14 oz) coconut milk
- 2 tablespoons curry powder
- 1 teaspoon ground turmeric
- 1 teaspoon ground cumin
- 1 teaspoon ground coriander
- 1/2 teaspoon red pepper flakes (optional)
- Salt and pepper to taste
- Fresh cilantro leaves for garnish (optional)
- Cooked rice or naan bread for serving

Instructions:

1. Heat the olive oil in a big saucepan or Dutch oven over medium heat.
2. Add the diced onion to the saucepan and cook it for two to three minutes, or until it becomes soft.
3. Add the grated ginger and minced garlic, stirring, and simmer for an additional minute, or until fragrant.

4. Include the bell pepper, zucchini, and chopped carrots in the saucepan. Cook, stirring occasionally, until the veggies are slightly cooked, 5 to 7 minutes.
5. Add the chopped tomatoes with their juices, coconut milk, and rinsed and drained lentils.
6. Add the red pepper flakes (if using), curry powder, ground turmeric, ground cumin, and ground coriander. To taste, add salt and pepper for seasoning.
7. Bring the mixture to a simmer, cover, lower the heat, and cook for 20 to 25 minutes, or until the veggies and lentils are soft and the curry has somewhat thickened.
8. Taste and, if necessary, adjust seasoning.
9. **Optional:** Before serving, sprinkle some fresh cilantro leaves over the lentil and vegetable curry.
10. Serve hot with naan bread on the side or over cooked rice.

18. Zesty Shrimp and Quinoa Salad

Ingredients:

For the Shrimp:

- 1 lb large shrimp, peeled and deveined
- 2 tablespoons olive oil
- 1 teaspoon smoked paprika

- 1 teaspoon cumin
- 1/2 teaspoon garlic powder
- Salt and pepper to taste
- Zest of 1 lemon

For the Quinoa Salad:

- 1 cup quinoa, rinsed
- 2 cups water or vegetable broth
- 1 cup cherry tomatoes, halved
- 1 cucumber, diced
- 1/4 cup red onion, finely chopped
- 1/4 cup fresh cilantro, chopped
- Juice of 1 lemon
- 2 tablespoons olive oil
- Salt and pepper to taste
- Avocado slices for garnish (optional)

Instructions:

For the Shrimp:

1. Combine olive oil, cumin, garlic powder, smoked paprika, salt, pepper, and lemon zest in a bowl.
2. Include the shrimp in the bowl once they have been peeled and deveined, and toss to coat with marinade. Give them ten to fifteen minutes to marinade.

3. Cook the marinated shrimp in a pan over medium-high heat for two to three minutes on each side, or until they become opaque and pink. Put aside.

For the Quinoa Salad:

1. Put the quinoa, water or vegetable broth, and a small amount of salt in a pot. After bringing to a boil, lower the heat to a simmer, cover, and cook the quinoa for approximately fifteen minutes, or until the water has been absorbed.
2. Put the cooked quinoa, sliced cucumber, chopped red onion, cherry tomatoes, and fresh cilantro in a big bowl.
3. Combine the lemon juice, olive oil, salt, and pepper in a small bowl. After adding the dressing, toss the quinoa salad to mix it well.
4. Place the cooked shrimp on top of the quinoa salad.
5. You can choose to add avocado slices as a garnish.

19. Tomato Basil Grilled Eggplant

Ingredients:

- 1 large eggplant, sliced into 1/2-inch rounds

- 2 tablespoons olive oil
- Salt and pepper to taste
- 2 large tomatoes, sliced
- 1/4 cup fresh basil leaves
- 2 cloves garlic, minced
- 1/4 cup grated Parmesan cheese (optional)
- Balsamic glaze for drizzling (optional)

Instructions:

1. Turn the heat up to medium-high on your grill or grill pan.
2. Season the eggplant slices with salt and pepper after rubbing them with olive oil on both sides.
3. Grill the eggplant slices for three to four minutes on each side, or until they are soft and have grill marks.
4. Make the tomato-basil topping while the eggplant is roasting. Sliced tomatoes, fresh basil leaves, minced garlic, and a splash of olive oil should all be combined in a small bowl. To taste, add salt and pepper for seasoning.
5. After the eggplant slices are cooked, take them off the grill and put them on a dish for serving.
6. Place a dollop of the tomato-basil mixture over each cooked eggplant slice.
7. Optional: For added taste, sprinkle with grated Parmesan cheese.

8. For a sweet and tangy touch, drizzle some balsamic sauce over the grilled eggplant with tomato and basil.

9. Serve hot and savor this flavorful and nourishing meal.

20. Cauliflower Fried Rice with Tofu

Ingredients:

- 1 head cauliflower, riced (or about 4 cups cauliflower rice)
- 1 tablespoon sesame oil
- 2 tablespoons soy sauce (or tamari for gluten-free option)
- 2 cloves garlic, minced
- 1 tablespoon grated ginger
- 1 block extra firm tofu, pressed and diced
- 1 cup mixed vegetables (such as carrots, peas, corn, and bell peppers)
- 2 green onions, sliced
- 2 eggs, beaten (optional)
- Salt and pepper to taste
- Sesame seeds and sliced green onions for garnish

Instructions:

1. In a food processor, pulse the cauliflower florets until they resemble rice grains to make the cauliflower rice. You may also use prepackaged cauliflower rice.

2. Heat the sesame oil in a big skillet or wok over medium heat.

3. Add the grated ginger and minced garlic to the skillet and cook for one to two minutes, or until fragrant.

4. Add the diced tofu to the skillet and heat, turning periodically, until the tofu is gently browned, about 5 to 7 minutes.

5. Transfer the mixed veggies to one side of the pan and push the tofu to the other. Simmer the veggies for 3–4 minutes, or until they are soft.

6. Push the veggies and tofu to one side of the skillet and fill the empty space with the beaten eggs. After the eggs are fully cooked, stir them into the tofu and veggies.

7. Add the cauliflower rice to the skillet along with the eggs, veggies, and tofu, and mix to incorporate.

8. To ensure that everything is properly coated, drizzle soy sauce (or tamari) over the cauliflower rice mixture and toss.

9. Cook the cauliflower rice for five to seven minutes, stirring now and again, until it's soft and well cooked.

10. Add pepper and salt to taste.

11. Optional: Before serving, garnish with sliced green onions and sesame seeds.

CHAPTER FIVE: SNACKS AND APPETIZERS FOR HEART HEALTH

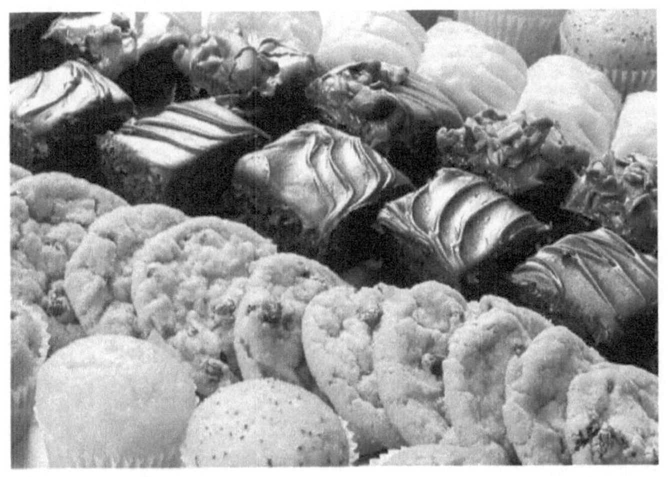

1. Cucumber and Hummus Bites

Ingredients:

- 1 large cucumber
- Hummus (store-bought or homemade)
- Cherry tomatoes, sliced (optional)
- Black olives, sliced (optional)
- Fresh parsley or dill for garnish (optional)

Instructions:

1. Give the cucumber a good wash and use paper towels to pat dry.
2. Cut the cucumber into rounds that are around half an inch thick.
3. To make a little well for the hummus, you can, if you'd like, use a miniature spoon or melon baller to scoop out a small depression in the middle of each cucumber slice.
4. Place a little dollop of hummus onto every slice of cucumber.
5. **Optional:** For extra taste and appearance, top each cucumber and hummus bite with a cherry tomato slice, a black olive slice, or a sprig of fresh parsley or dill.
6. Transfer the cucumber and hummus morsels to a dish for presentation.
7. Serve right away as a wholesome and revitalizing snack or appetizer.

2. Mixed Nuts and Seeds Trail Mix

Ingredients:

- 1 cup almonds
- 1 cup cashews
- 1 cup walnuts
- 1/2 cup pumpkin seeds (pepitas)
- 1/2 cup sunflower seeds
- 1/4 cup dried cranberries
- 1/4 cup raisins
- 1/4 cup dried apricots, chopped
- 1/4 cup dark chocolate chips (optional)
- 1 teaspoon cinnamon (optional)
- 1/2 teaspoon sea salt (optional)

Instructions:

1. Place the almonds, cashews, walnuts, pumpkin seeds, and sunflower seeds in a large mixing basin.
2. Fill the bowl with the chopped dried apricots, raisins, dried cranberries, and dark chocolate chips (if using).
3. For added taste, you may top the mixture with sea salt and cinnamon, if you'd like.
4. Combine everything and toss until thoroughly mixed.
5. To make it simple to munch on the move, transfer the mixed nuts and seeds trail mix to an airtight

container or separate it into individual, portion-sized bags.

6. Trail mix can be kept for up to two weeks in a cool, dry location.

You may alter this recipe for trail mix by substituting your preferred dried fruits, nuts, or seeds for any of the ingredients. For variation, you may also add other items like dried pineapple, pretzel bits, or coconut flakes.

3. Mango Salsa with Shrimp

Ingredients:

For the Mango Salsa:

- 2 ripe mangoes, peeled, pitted, and diced
- 1/2 red onion, finely chopped
- 1 red bell pepper, diced
- 1 jalapeño, seeds removed and finely chopped
- 1/4 cup fresh cilantro, chopped
- Juice of 2 limes
- Salt and pepper to taste

For the Shrimp:

- 1 lb large shrimp, peeled and deveined

- 1 tablespoon olive oil
- 1 teaspoon smoked paprika
- 1/2 teaspoon cumin
- Salt and pepper to taste
- Lime wedges for serving

Instructions:

For the Mango Salsa:

1. Combine diced mangoes, lime juice, salt, and pepper in a bowl with finely sliced red onion, diced red bell pepper, chopped jalapeño, and chopped fresh cilantro. Blend well.

2. As you're making the shrimp, adjust the spice to taste and chill the mango salsa.

For the Shrimp:

1. Combine olive oil, cumin, smoked paprika, salt, and pepper in a bowl.

2. Make sure the peeled and deveined shrimp are equally covered by tossing them in the spice mixture.

3. Cook the seasoned shrimp in a pan over medium-high heat for two to three minutes on each side, or until they become opaque and pink.

4. Transfer the cooked shrimp to a platter and top with the cool mango salsa.

5. You may optionally add more cilantro and lime wedges as garnish.

4. *Whole Grain Crackers with Avocado*

Ingredients:

- Whole grain crackers
- 2 ripe avocados
- Cherry tomatoes, sliced (optional)
- Red pepper flakes (optional)
- Lemon juice
- Salt and pepper to taste

Instructions:

1. Scoop the avocado flesh into a dish after cutting the avocados in half and removing the seeds.
2. Using a fork, mash the avocado until the appropriate consistency is reached.
3. To add brightness and stop the mashed avocado from browning, squeeze fresh lemon juice over it.
4. To taste, add salt and pepper to the mashed avocado. If you would want a little kick of heat, you may also add a pinch of red pepper flakes.
5. Cover whole grain crackers with avocado mash.

6. You may optionally add sliced cherry tomatoes on the top of each cracker to add more freshness.

5. *Roasted Chickpeas Snack*

Ingredients:

- 2 cans (15 oz each) chickpeas (garbanzo beans), drained and rinsed
- 2 tablespoons olive oil
- 1 teaspoon ground cumin
- 1 teaspoon smoked paprika
- 1/2 teaspoon garlic powder
- 1/2 teaspoon onion powder
- 1/4 teaspoon cayenne pepper (optional, for heat)
- Salt to taste

Instructions:

1. Set the oven temperature to 400°F, or 200°C. For easier cleanup, line a baking pan with aluminum foil or parchment paper.
2. After the chickpeas have been rinsed and drained, spread them out on a fresh kitchen towel and pat dry. Eliminate any fallen skin that becomes loose.
3. Toss the dry chickpeas with olive oil in a big mixing basin until they are well covered.

4. Combine the ground cumin, smoked paprika, onion and garlic powders, salt, and cayenne pepper (if using) in a small bowl.

5. Distribute the spice blend onto the chickpeas and stir until they are thoroughly coated.

6. Arrange the seasoned chickpeas on the baking sheet that has been prepared in a single layer.

7. Roast the chickpeas for 20 to 30 minutes in a preheated oven, stirring the pan halfway through, or until they are crispy and browned.

8. After roasting, take the chickpeas out of the oven and let them cool for a short while on the baking sheet.

9. To enjoy the roasted chickpeas later, serve them warm as a snack or let them cool fully before putting them in an airtight container.

6. Smoked Salmon Cucumber Rounds

Ingredients:

- English cucumbers, sliced into rounds
- Smoked salmon, thinly sliced
- Cream cheese or Greek yogurt
- Fresh dill, chopped
- Lemon zest
- Capers (optional)
- Black pepper

Instructions:

1. Cut the English cucumbers into rounds that range in thickness from 1/4 to 1/2 inch.
2. Top each cucumber circle with a little dollop of cream cheese or Greek yogurt.
3. Arrange a smoked salmon slice over the yogurt or cream cheese.
4. Top the smoked salmon with freshly chopped dill.
5. For added freshness, sprinkle some lemon zest on top of each round.
6. You may add capers as an optional garnish to add some flavor.
7. Add a dash of black pepper to finish.

Place your Smoked Salmon Cucumber Rounds on a tray, then savor this sophisticated and delicious snack or appetizer!

7. Guacamole with Veggie Sticks

Ingredients:

For the Guacamole:

- 2 ripe avocados

- 1 small tomato, diced
- 1/4 cup red onion, finely chopped
- 1 jalapeño pepper, seeded and finely chopped (optional)
- 1-2 tablespoons fresh lime juice
- 2 tablespoons fresh cilantro, chopped
- Salt and pepper to taste

For the Veggie Sticks:

- Carrot sticks
- Cucumber sticks
- Bell pepper strips
- Celery sticks

Instructions:

For the Guacamole:

1. Remove the pits from the avocados by cutting them in half lengthwise. Remove the meat and transfer it to a medium-sized bowl.
2. Mash the avocado with a fork until it's smooth or the consistency you want.
3. Combine the mashed avocado with diced tomato, finely chopped red onion, jalapeño pepper (if using), fresh lime juice, and chopped cilantro in a bowl.
4. To taste, add salt and pepper for seasoning.

5. Gently mix everything until thoroughly blended.
6. If necessary, taste and adjust the seasoning. To adjust for acidity, add extra lime juice and/or salt and pepper to taste.
7. Refrigerate the guacamole until it's time to serve by covering it with plastic wrap and pressing it firmly onto the guacamole's surface to avoid browning.

For the Veggie Sticks:

1. Clean and slice the bell pepper, celery, cucumber, and carrots into sticks or strips.
2. Place the veggie sticks in separate containers or on a serving dish.

To Serve:

1. Present the veggie sticks with the chilled guacamole.
2. Savor the delicious and creamy guacamole dipped in the crunchy veggie sticks!

8. Caprese Skewers with Balsamic Glaze

Ingredients:

- Cherry tomatoes
- Fresh mozzarella balls (or mozzarella cut into bite-sized pieces)
- Fresh basil leaves
- Balsamic glaze
- Wooden or metal skewers

Instructions:

1. Wash and cut in half the cherry tomatoes to prepare them.
2. Chop fresh mozzarella into bite-sized pieces if you're not using premade balls.
3. Take a skewer and put a cherry tomato, a basil leaf, and a mozzarella slice on it. Continue until all the skewers are filled..
4. Put the caprese skewers on a plate for serving.
5. Drizzle the skewers with balsamic glaze.
6. For more taste, feel free to add a small pinch of salt and pepper.

Present your Balsamic Glazed Caprese Skewers as a bright and wonderful appetizer or snack!

9. Walnut and Grape Bruschetta

Ingredients:

- 1 French baguette, sliced into 1/2-inch thick rounds
- 1 cup red seedless grapes, halved
- 1/2 cup walnuts, chopped
- 4 ounces goat cheese
- Honey, for drizzling
- Fresh thyme leaves, for garnish
- Olive oil, for drizzling
- Salt and pepper to taste

Instructions:

1. Set the oven temperature to 375°F, or 190°C.
2. Arrange the baguette slices on an oven tray and gently mist them with olive oil. Add a dash of pepper and salt for seasoning.
3. Toast the baguette slices for 8 to 10 minutes, or until they are crisp and gently brown.
4. Combine the chopped walnuts and the half-grapes in a small bowl.
5. Top each piece of toasted bread with a heaping tablespoon of goat cheese.
6. Place a layer of the grape and walnut mixture on top of each baguette slice, carefully pressing it in place.
7. For a hint of sweetness, drizzle honey over the top of each bruschetta.

8. Add some fresh thyme leaves to the walnut and grape bruschetta as a garnish.
9. Serve as a snack or appetizer right away.

10. Edamame and Sesame Seed Salad

Ingredients:

- 2 cups shelled edamame (frozen, thawed)
- 1 cup red cabbage, thinly sliced
- 1 cup carrots, julienned or grated
- 1/4 cup green onions, sliced
- 2 tablespoons sesame seeds (toasted for extra flavor)
- 3 tablespoons soy sauce
- 2 tablespoons rice vinegar
- 1 tablespoon sesame oil
- 1 tablespoon honey or maple syrup
- 1 teaspoon fresh ginger, grated
- 1 clove garlic, minced
- Salt and pepper to taste

Instructions:

1. Combine sliced red cabbage, sliced green onions, julienned or shredded carrots, shelled edamame, and sesame seeds in a big bowl.

2. Combine the soy sauce, rice vinegar, sesame oil, honey or maple syrup, chopped garlic, grated fresh ginger, salt, and pepper in a different small bowl. To suit your tastes, adjust the sweetness and saltiness.

3. Drizzle the edamame and veggie combination with the dressing. In order to coat everything equally, toss well.

4. To enable the flavors to mingle, let the salad marinade in the fridge for at least 15 to 20 minutes.

5. Before serving, feel free to top with more sesame seeds and green onions.

11. Zucchini Fritters with Yogurt Sauce

Ingredients:

For the Zucchini Fritters:

- 2 medium zucchinis
- 1 teaspoon salt
- 2 eggs
- 1/4 cup grated Parmesan cheese
- 1/4 cup all-purpose flour or almond flour (for gluten-free option)
- 2 cloves garlic, minced
- 2 tablespoons chopped fresh parsley or dill

- 1/2 teaspoon black pepper
- Olive oil for frying

For the Yogurt Sauce:

- 1/2 cup Greek yogurt
- 1 tablespoon lemon juice
- 1 tablespoon chopped fresh dill
- Salt and pepper to taste

Instructions:

For the Zucchini Fritters:

1. Using a food processor or box grater, finely chop the zucchini. To remove extra moisture, put the shredded zucchini in a sieve, season with salt, and let sit for about ten minutes.
2. After ten minutes, squeeze as much liquid out of the shredded zucchini as you can using your hands or a fresh kitchen towel.
3. Add the grated zucchini, eggs, Parmesan cheese, flour, minced garlic, chopped fresh parsley or dill, and black pepper to a large mixing bowl. Blend until well blended.
4. In a big skillet over medium heat, add a thin coating of olive oil.
5. Using the back of a spoon, gently press spoonfuls of the zucchini mixture into the pan.

6. Fry the fritters for three to four minutes on each side, or until crispy and golden brown. The size of your skillet will determine whether you need to work in batches.

7. After cooking, move the fritters to a platter covered with paper towels so that any extra oil may be drained off.

For the Yogurt Sauce:

1. In a small bowl, mix together the Greek yogurt, lemon juice, chopped fresh dill, salt, and pepper until well combined.

2. Taste and adjust seasoning if needed.

To Serve:

1. Present the warm zucchini fritters beside a dish of yogurt sauce for dipping.

2. If preferred, garnish with more finely chopped fresh herbs.

3. Savor these tasty and crispy fritters as an appetizer!

12. Vegetable Spring Rolls with Peanut Dipping Sauce

Ingredients:

For Vegetable Spring Rolls:

- Rice paper wrappers
- 1 cup rice vermicelli noodles, cooked and cooled
- 1 cup lettuce, shredded
- 1 cup carrots, julienned
- 1 cup cucumber, julienned
- 1/2 cup red bell pepper, julienned
- Fresh mint leaves
- Fresh cilantro leaves
- Cooked and sliced tofu or shrimp (optional)

For Peanut Dipping Sauce:

- 1/4 cup peanut butter
- 2 tablespoons soy sauce
- 1 tablespoon rice vinegar
- 1 tablespoon honey or maple syrup
- 1 teaspoon sesame oil
- 1 clove garlic, minced
- Water (to thin the sauce)
- Crushed peanuts for garnish (optional)

Instructions:

For Vegetable Spring Rolls:

1. Get all the veggies ready for assembly by preparing them beforehand.

2. Pour warm water into a large shallow dish. For five to ten seconds, dip one rice paper wrapper into the water until it becomes flexible but not too soft.

3. Lay the damp rice paper out on a dish towel or a sanitized surface.

4. Arrange a little amount of cooked rice vermicelli noodles, cucumber, red bell pepper, shredded lettuce, julienned carrots, and a few fresh cilantro and mint leaves in the center of the rice paper.

5. You may add cooked tofu or shrimp pieces if you'd like.

6. Tightly twist the rice paper into a spring roll by folding the sides over the filling and then the bottom.

7. Continue using the remaining components.

For Peanut Dipping Sauce:

1. Combine peanut butter, soy sauce, rice vinegar, sesame oil, honey or maple syrup, and chopped garlic in a bowl.

2. Gradually add water to get the consistency of the dipping sauce that you want.

3. You might choose to add crushed peanuts as a garnish.

Serve the Peanut Dipping Sauce alongside the Vegetable Spring Rolls, and savor this tasty and refreshing treat!

13. Artichoke and Spinach Dip with Whole Wheat Pita

Ingredients:

For the Artichoke and Spinach Dip:

- 1 (10 oz) package frozen chopped spinach, thawed and drained
- 1 (14 oz) can artichoke hearts, drained and chopped
- 1 cup shredded mozzarella cheese
- 1/2 cup grated Parmesan cheese
- 1/2 cup plain Greek yogurt
- 1/4 cup mayonnaise
- 2 cloves garlic, minced
- 1 teaspoon dried basil
- 1/2 teaspoon dried oregano
- Salt and pepper to taste

For Serving:

- Whole wheat pita bread, cut into wedges

- Fresh vegetables for dipping (carrot sticks, cucumber slices, bell pepper strips, etc.)

Instructions:

1. Set the oven temperature to 375°F, or 190°C.
2. Add the chopped spinach, chopped artichoke hearts, grated Parmesan cheese, shredded mozzarella cheese, Greek yogurt, mayonnaise, minced garlic, dried oregano, dried basil, and salt and pepper to a large mixing bowl. Blend until well blended.
3. Spoon the mixture into an oven-safe pan or baking dish that has been oiled.
4. Bake for 25 to 30 minutes in a preheated oven, or until the top of the dip is bubbling and golden brown.
5. Cut the whole wheat pita bread into wedges and prepare while the dip bakes.
6. Take the dip out of the oven and allow it to cool a little before serving.
7. Present the warm Spinach and Artichoke Dip alongside fresh veggies for dipping and whole wheat pita wedges.

14. Quinoa Stuffed Mushrooms

Ingredients:

- 1 cup quinoa, cooked
- 20-25 large mushrooms, cleaned and stems removed
- 1 tablespoon olive oil
- 1 small onion, finely chopped
- 2 cloves garlic, minced
- 1 cup spinach, chopped
- 1/4 cup sun-dried tomatoes, chopped
- 1/4 cup feta cheese, crumbled
- 1/4 cup grated Parmesan cheese
- 1 teaspoon dried oregano
- Salt and pepper to taste
- Fresh parsley for garnish (optional)

Instructions:

1. Set the oven temperature to 375°F, or 190°C.
2. Prepare the quinoa per the directions on the package and set it aside.
3. Heat the olive oil in a pan over medium heat. Add the chopped onion and garlic, and cook until they become soft.
4. Cook the chopped spinach in the pan until it wilts.
5. Add the cooked quinoa, feta cheese, and sun-dried tomatoes. Simmer for a further two to

three minutes to let the flavors combine. Add salt, pepper, and dried oregano for seasoning.

6. Turn off the heat on the skillet.

7. Gently push the quinoa mixture into each of the mushroom caps.

8. Transfer the filled mushrooms to an ovenproof sheet.

9. Top each filled mushroom with a grating of Parmesan cheese.

10. Bake the mushrooms for 15 to 20 minutes, or until they are soft, in a preheated oven.

11. Before serving, you may optionally garnish with fresh parsley.

Savor the taste and nutritional value of your Quinoa Stuffed Mushrooms appetizer.

15. Dark Chocolate-Dipped Strawberries

Ingredients:

- Fresh strawberries, washed and dried
- Dark chocolate chips or chopped dark chocolate (at least 70% cocoa)
- Optional toppings: chopped nuts, shredded coconut, sprinkles, sea salt flakes, etc.

Instructions:

1. Use wax or parchment paper to line a baking pan.
2. Melt the chopped dark chocolate or dark chocolate chips in a heatproof dish over a double boiler or in the microwave for 30-second bursts, stirring until smooth.

Grasping each strawberry by its stem, submerge it into the liquefied chocolate, rotating it to cover approximately two-thirds of the fruit.

4. After letting any extra chocolate drip off, put the strawberry that has been dipped onto the baking sheet that has been ready.
5. While the chocolate is still wet, sprinkle your preferred toppings over the strawberries that have been dipped.
6. Use the remaining strawberries to repeat the dipping procedure.
7. Refrigerate the baking sheet for fifteen to twenty minutes, or until the chocolate sets.
8. After the dark chocolate-dipped strawberries have hardened, move them to a dish or plate.
9. Serve right away as a tasty treat or dessert.

CHAPTER SIX: SATISFYING DESSERTS THAT LOVE YOUR HEART

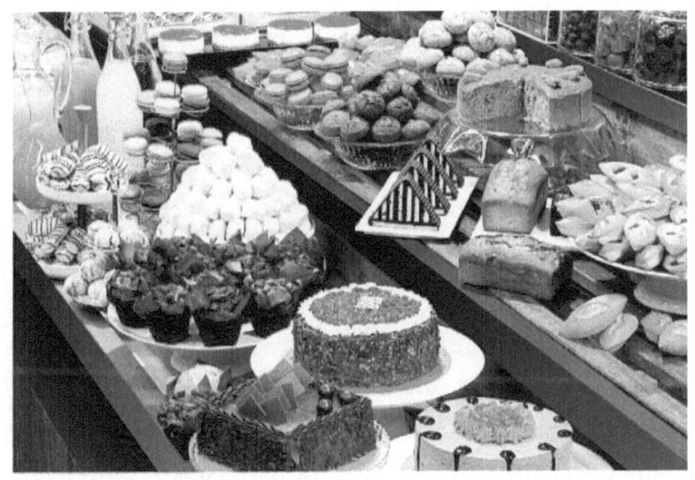

1. Orange Dark Chocolate Truffles

Ingredients:

- 8 oz (about 1 1/3 cups) dark chocolate, finely chopped
- 1/2 cup heavy cream
- Zest of 1 orange
- 2 tablespoons unsalted butter, softened
- Cocoa powder or finely chopped nuts for coating (optional)

Instructions:

1. Place the heavy cream in a saucepan and boil over medium heat until it begins to simmer.
2. Fill a heatproof basin with the finely chopped dark chocolate.
3. Cover the chocolate with the heated cream, then wait a minute for the chocolate to melt.
4. Blend the chocolate and cream blend until it's smooth and well mixed.
5. Include the orange zest and melted butter in the chocolate mixture. Mix the ingredients until it becomes smooth and the butter has melted.
6. Once the mixture is hard enough to handle, cover the bowl and refrigerate it for at least two hours.
7. After the chocolate mixture solidifies, scoop out parts with a spoon or melon baller and form them into little balls.
8. You can choose to cover the truffles with cocoa powder or finely chopped almonds.

9. To set, place the coated truffles on a tray covered with parchment paper and refrigerate for a further half hour.

10. Until you're ready to serve, keep the orange dark chocolate truffles in the refrigerator in an airtight container.

2. *Avocado Chocolate Mousse*

Ingredients:

- 2 ripe avocados
- 1/4 cup cocoa powder
- 1/4 cup maple syrup or honey
- 1 teaspoon vanilla extract
- Pinch of salt
- **Optional toppings**: whipped cream, berries, shaved chocolate, chopped nuts

Instructions:

1. Halve the avocados, remove the pits, and transfer the flesh to a food processor or blender.

2. Fill the blender or food processor with cocoa powder, vanilla extract, maple syrup or honey, and a dash of salt.

3. Blend, scraping down the sides as necessary to ensure everything is fully blended, until the mixture is smooth and creamy.

4. Taste the avocado chocolate mousse and, if required, reduce the sweetness or add more cocoa powder.

5. Spoon the mousse into glasses or serving dishes.

6. To let the flavors combine and the mouse cool, cover and chill in the refrigerator for a minimum of half an hour.

7. You may add whipped cream, berries, shaved chocolate, chopped nuts, or any other toppings you choose to the avocado chocolate mousse before serving.

8. Enjoy this rich and creamy delight while it's cooled!

3. Coconut Bliss Balls

Ingredients:

- 1 cup shredded coconut (plus extra for coating)
- 1 cup Medjool dates, pitted
- 1/2 cup raw almonds
- 2 tablespoons coconut oil, melted
- 1 teaspoon vanilla extract
- Pinch of salt

Instructions:

1. Grated coconut, pitted Medjool dates, raw almonds, melted coconut oil, vanilla essence, and a dash of salt should all be combined in a food processor.
2. Put the ingredients through a food processor until a uniformly sticky dough is formed.
3. Scoop out little bits of dough and roll them in your palms to create bliss balls the size of bites.
4. To coat the outside, if preferred, roll each bliss ball in more shredded coconut.
5. Transfer the coconut bliss balls to a dish lined with parchment paper and chill for a minimum of half an hour to solidify.
6. The bliss balls can be savored once they've chilled.

4. Pumpkin Spice Oat Cookies

Ingredients:

- 1 cup rolled oats
- 1 cup all-purpose flour or whole wheat flour
- 1/2 teaspoon baking soda
- 1/2 teaspoon baking powder
- 1 teaspoon ground cinnamon
- 1/2 teaspoon ground ginger

- 1/4 teaspoon ground nutmeg
- 1/4 teaspoon ground cloves
- 1/4 teaspoon salt
- 1/2 cup unsalted butter, softened
- 1/2 cup granulated sugar
- 1/2 cup packed brown sugar
- 1 egg
- 1 teaspoon vanilla extract
- 3/4 cup pumpkin puree
- 1/2 cup raisins or chopped nuts (optional)

Instructions:

1. Set the oven temperature to 175°C, or 350°F. Use silicone baking mats or parchment paper to line a baking pan.
2. In a medium-sized mixing bowl, thoroughly mix the flour, baking powder, baking soda, nutmeg, cloves, cinnamon, ginger, and salt.
3. Using a large mixing basin, beat the brown sugar, granulated sugar, and melted butter until creamy and light.
4. Until smooth, beat in the egg and vanilla extract.
5. Ensure that the pumpkin puree is well mixed in.
6. Mix until just incorporated, gradually add the dry ingredients to the wet components. Take caution not to blend too much.
7. If using, mix the chopped nuts or raisins into the cookie mixture until they are spread evenly.

8. Leaving room between each cookie for spreading, drop spoonfuls of the cookie dough onto the baking sheet that has been prepared.

9. Using the back of a spoon or fork, gently flatten each cookie.

10. Bake for 10 to 12 minutes, or until the sides are just beginning to turn golden brown, in a preheated oven.

11. Take the cookies out of the oven and allow them to rest for a few minutes on the baking sheet, then move them to a wire rack to cool down fully.

12. Serve and savor these delectable Pumpkin Spice Oat Cookies when they've cooled!

5. Mixed Berry Frozen Yogurt Pops

Ingredients:

- 1 cup mixed berries (strawberries, blueberries, raspberries), fresh or frozen
- 2 cups Greek yogurt
- 1/4 cup honey or maple syrup
- 1 teaspoon vanilla extract

Instructions:

1. Place mixed berries, Greek yogurt, honey (or maple syrup), and vanilla extract in a blender or food processor.
2. Puree the mixture until it's smooth and well mixed.
3. Fill popsicle molds with the berry yogurt mixture, allowing a small space at the top for expansion.
4. Place the popsicle sticks inside the molds.
5. Freeze the popsicles for four to six hours, or until they are fully set.
6. To extract the popsicles from the molds once they have frozen, briefly submerge them in warm water.
7. Savor your tasty frozen yogurt pops with mixed berries!

6. Walnut Date Bars

Ingredients:

- 1 cup pitted dates
- 1 cup walnuts
- 1/2 cup rolled oats
- 1/4 cup shredded coconut
- 1 tablespoon coconut oil, melted
- 1 teaspoon vanilla extract
- Pinch of salt

Instructions:

1. Set the oven temperature to 175°C, or 350°F. An 8x8-inch baking dish should be greased or lined with parchment paper.

2. Put the shredded coconut, rolled oats, melted coconut oil, vanilla essence, pitted dates, and a dash of salt in a food processor.

3. Pulse the ingredients until everything is fully incorporated and the mixture resembles sticky dough. You can add another tablespoon of melted coconut oil or water if the mixture appears too dry.

4. Using a spatula or your hands, transfer the mixture to the baking dish that has been prepared and press it firmly and evenly into the bottom.

5. Bake for 15 to 18 minutes, or until the edges are golden brown, in an oven that has been prepared.

6. Take out of the oven and let the baked dish cool fully before slicing into bars.

7. Using a sharp knife, cut into bars or squares when it has cooled.

8. To maintain freshness for a longer period of time, store the walnut date bars in the refrigerator or at room temperature in an airtight container for up to a week.

7. Cherry Almond Yogurt Parfait

Ingredients:

- 1 cup Greek yogurt
- 1 cup fresh or frozen cherries, pitted and halved
- 1/4 cup almonds, sliced or chopped
- 2 tablespoons honey or maple syrup
- 1/2 teaspoon almond extract (optional)
- Granola for layering (optional)

Instructions:

1. Combine Greek yogurt and honey or maple syrup in a bowl. Add some almond extract for taste if you'd like.

2. Arrange the Greek yogurt mixture in dishes or glasses and top with frozen or fresh cherries.

3. Top each layer with sliced or chopped almonds.

4. You may optionally top with granola for extra texture and crunch.

5. Continue layering until all of the bowls or glasses are full.

6. Add a little more almond slices and a drizzle of honey or maple syrup to the parfait to finish it off.

7. Present your Cherry Almond Yogurt Parfait promptly and savor it!

8. Dark Chocolate-Dipped Bananas

Ingredients:

- 2 ripe bananas
- 4 ounces dark chocolate (at least 70% cocoa), chopped
- 1 tablespoon coconut oil or vegetable oil
- Optional toppings: chopped nuts, shredded coconut, sprinkles, sea salt flakes

Instructions:

1. After peeling, split the bananas in half lengthwise. If you want to make the banana halves easier to handle, insert a popsicle stick into each one.
2. Use parchment paper to line a baking sheet.
3. In a dish that is microwave-safe, combine the chopped dark chocolate and coconut oil.
4. Microwave the chocolate until it melts and becomes smooth, stirring every 30 seconds.
5. Using a spoon or spatula to help coat them equally, dip each half of a banana into the melted chocolate.
6. After letting any extra chocolate drip off, put the bananas that have been dipped in chocolate onto the baking sheet that has been ready.
7. While the chocolate is still wet, top the bananas that have been dipped in chocolate, if you'd like.

8. After dipping and decorating all of the bananas, chill the baking sheet in the fridge for fifteen to twenty minutes, or until the chocolate sets.

9. When the dark chocolate-dipped bananas have set, take them out of the refrigerator and serve right away. Alternatively, you may put them in the fridge in an airtight container to enjoy them later.

9. Baked Apple with Cinnamon and Walnuts

Ingredients:

- 2 apples (such as Granny Smith or Honeycrisp)
- 2 tablespoons chopped walnuts
- 1 tablespoon honey or maple syrup
- 1 teaspoon ground cinnamon
- 1 tablespoon unsalted butter, melted
- Vanilla ice cream or yogurt for serving (optional)

Instructions:

1. Set the oven temperature to 375°F, or 190°C.

2. To make a well for the filling, wash and core the apples, being careful to leave the bottoms intact.

3. Combine ground cinnamon, honey or maple syrup, and chopped walnuts in a small bowl.

4. Transfer the apple cores to a baking tray.

5. Stuff the combination of walnuts and cinnamon inside each apple.

6. Top each filled apple with a drizzle of melted butter.

7. Bake the apples for 25 to 30 minutes, or until they are soft, in a preheated oven.

8. You might choose to drizzle the apples with some of the baking dish's juices midway through baking.

9. After baking, take the apples out of the oven and give them a little time to cool.

10. If preferred, top the baked apples with a dollop of yogurt or a scoop of vanilla ice cream.

10. Mango Sorbet with Mint

Ingredients:

- 4 ripe mangoes, peeled, pitted, and diced
- 1/2 cup granulated sugar (adjust to taste, depending on the sweetness of the mangoes)
- 1/4 cup water
- 2 tablespoons fresh lime juice
- Fresh mint leaves for garnish

Instructions:

1. Place the water and granulated sugar in a small saucepan. Stirring periodically, cook over medium heat until the sugar dissolves completely. After taking off the heat, allow the simple syrup to reach room temperature.

2. Place the chopped mangoes, cooled simple syrup, and fresh lime juice in a food processor or blender.

3. Blend until creamy and smooth, stopping occasionally to scrape down the sides of the food processor or blender.

4. Taste the mixture and, if needed, add additional sugar or lime juice to balance the sweetness or sharpness.

5. Pour the mango mixture into an ice cream machine and process, following the manufacturer's directions, until the consistency of the mixture resembles sorbet.

6. You may transfer the mango mixture to a shallow dish and freeze it if you don't have an ice cream machine. Use a fork to scrape and stir the mixture every 30 minutes until it gets solid and scoopable, which should take around 4-6 hours.

7. Spoon the mango sorbet into glasses or serving bowls as soon as it's done.

8. Before serving, garnish with fresh mint leaves.

9. Enjoy the cool, tropical tastes of this Mango Sorbet with Mint as soon as you serve it!

11. Oatmeal Raisin Energy Bites

Ingredients:

- 1 cup old-fashioned rolled oats
- 1/2 cup almond butter or peanut butter
- 1/3 cup honey or maple syrup
- 1/2 cup raisins
- 1/2 cup ground flaxseed
- 1 teaspoon vanilla extract
- 1/2 teaspoon ground cinnamon
- A pinch of salt

Instructions:

1. Pinch of salt, ground flaxseed, ground cinnamon, almond butter or peanut butter, honey, maple syrup, raisins, and rolled oats should all be combined in a big dish.
2. Thoroughly stir the ingredients until they are properly blended.
3. To make handling the mixture simpler, refrigerate it for approximately half an hour.
4. Using your hands, form the mixture into bite-sized balls when it is cold.
5. The energy bites should be arranged on a tray covered with parchment paper.
6. To set, refrigerate the energy bites for a further half hour.

7. After the Oatmeal Raisin Energy Bites are set, move them to an airtight container and keep them chilled.

8. Savor these nutrient-dense, energy-packed nibbles as a light and satisfying snack!

12. Blueberry Chia Seed Smoothie Bowl

Ingredients:

- 1 ripe banana, frozen
- 1 cup frozen blueberries
- 1/2 cup Greek yogurt
- 1/2 cup almond milk (or any milk of your choice)
- 2 tablespoons chia seeds
- 1 tablespoon honey or maple syrup (optional, for added sweetness)
- **Toppings**: Fresh blueberries, sliced bananas, granola, shredded coconut, chia seeds, sliced almonds, or any other toppings of your choice

Instructions:

1. Put the frozen banana, Greek yogurt, frozen blueberries, almond milk, chia seeds, and honey or maple syrup (if using) in a blender.

2. Blend until creamy and smooth, adding extra almond milk as necessary to get the right consistency.

3. Transfer the blended drink to a bowl.

4. Top the smoothie bowl with the toppings of your choice.

5. Present right away and savor with a spoon!

13. Cocoa-Dusted Almonds

Ingredients:

- 1 cup whole almonds
- 1 tablespoon unsweetened cocoa powder
- 2 tablespoons powdered sugar
- 1/2 teaspoon vanilla extract
- A pinch of salt

Instructions:

1. Set the oven temperature to 175°C, or 350°F.

2. Toss the almonds until they are uniformly coated in a bowl with cocoa powder, powdered sugar, vanilla essence, and a little amount of salt.

3. Arrange the almonds coated in cocoa on a parchment paper-lined baking sheet.

4. Bake, stirring halfway through, for about 10 to 12 minutes in a preheated oven, or until the almonds are roasted and the cocoa coating sets.
5. Take the almonds out of the oven and allow them to cool fully.
6. Break apart any almonds that have bonded together once they have cooled.
7. Keep the cocoa-dusted almonds at room temperature in an airtight container.

14. Greek Yogurt and Honey Popsicles

Ingredients:

- 1 cup Greek yogurt
- 2 tablespoons honey (adjust to taste)
- 1 teaspoon vanilla extract (optional)
- Fresh berries, sliced fruit, or chopped nuts (optional)

Instructions:

1. Place the Greek yogurt, honey, and vanilla extract (if using) in a mixing bowl. Mix well until fully incorporated.
2. Taste the mixture and, if needed, add additional honey to balance the sweetness.

3. For extra texture and taste, gently stir in chopped nuts, sliced fruit, or fresh berries.

4. Fill each popsicle mold nearly to the brim with the yogurt mixture.

5. Place popsicle sticks in each mold's center.

6. To ensure that the mixture settles uniformly and to get rid of any air bubbles, lightly tap the molds on the tabletop.

7. After the popsicles are fully frozen, place the popsicle molds in the freezer and freeze for at least four to six hours.

8. After the popsicles have frozen, release them from the molds by briefly running warm water over their exterior.

9. Present the Greek yogurt and honey popsicles right away, then savor the smooth, sugary delight!

15. Lemon Blueberry Quinoa Cake

Ingredients:

For the Cake:

- 1 cup cooked quinoa, cooled
- 1 cup all-purpose flour
- 1 teaspoon baking powder
- 1/2 teaspoon baking soda
- 1/4 teaspoon salt

- Zest of 1 lemon
- 1/2 cup unsalted butter, softened
- 3/4 cup granulated sugar
- 2 large eggs
- 1 teaspoon vanilla extract
- 1/2 cup Greek yogurt
- 1 cup fresh or frozen blueberries

For the Lemon Glaze:

- 1 cup powdered sugar
- 2 tablespoons fresh lemon juice
- Zest of 1 lemon

Instructions:

For the Cake:

1. Set the oven temperature to 175°C, or 350°F. Butter and dust a 9-inch circular cake pan.
2. Combine the all-purpose flour, baking soda, baking powder, and salt in a medium-sized basin.
3. Transfer the cooked quinoa and lemon zest to another bowl.
4. In a different, sizable bowl, beat the granulated sugar and softened butter until they are frothy and light.
5. Beat thoroughly after adding each egg, one at a time. Add the vanilla essence and stir.

6. Alternately add the Greek yogurt and the dry components to the wet ingredients gradually. With the dry ingredients, start and finish.

7. Gently stir in the combination of quinoa and lemon zest.

8. Finally, mix the blueberries into the batter until they are uniformly distributed.

9. Transfer the mixture into the ready-made cake pan and level the surface.

10. Bake for about 35 to 40 minutes, or until a toothpick inserted in the middle comes out clean, in a preheated oven.

For the Lemon Glaze:

1. Combine the powdered sugar, lemon zest, and fresh lemon juice in a bowl and whisk until smooth.

2. After the cake cools, cover the top with the lemon glaze.

3. You may optionally add more lemon zest as a garnish.

Enjoy your delicious Lemon Blueberry Quinoa Cake after slicing it!

CHAPTER SEVEN: 7 DAY HEART-HEALTHY DELICIOUS MEAL PLAN

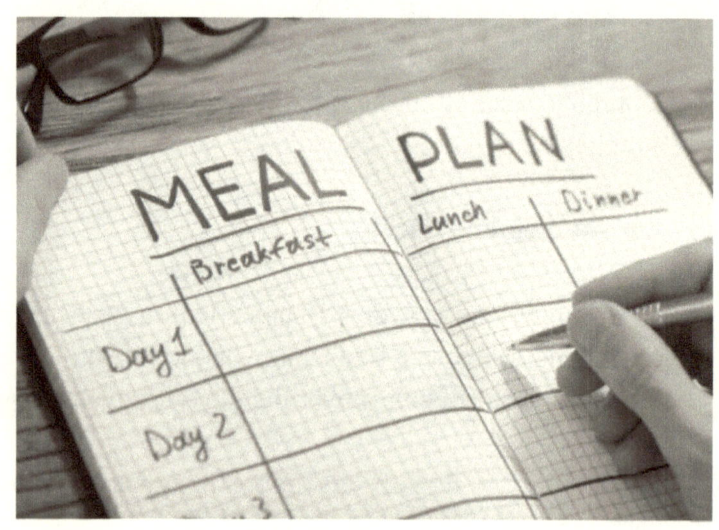

PLEASE NOTE THAT THIS IS A GENERAL PLAN, AND INDIVIDUAL DIETARY NEEDS MAY VARY

Day 1:

- Breakfast: Sweet Potato and Black Bean Breakfast Burrito

Ingredients:

- 1 large sweet potato, peeled and diced
- 1 can black beans, drained and rinsed
- 4 large eggs, scrambled
- Whole wheat or corn tortillas
- Avocado slices
- Salsa
- Fresh cilantro, chopped
- Olive oil for cooking
- Salt and pepper to taste

Instructions:

1. Heat the olive oil in a skillet over medium heat. Sweet potatoes should be added and sautéed until they are soft and start to caramelize.

2. Cook the sweet potatoes and drained black beans in a pan until they are well cooked.

3. Scramble the eggs in a different pan until they are cooked through. Add pepper and salt for seasoning.

4. Use a dry skillet or the microwave to reheat the tortillas.

5. Place some of the sweet potato and black bean mixture onto a tortilla to assemble the breakfast burritos.

6. Top with a few avocado slices, salsa, scrambled eggs, and fresh cilantro.

7. To make a burrito, fold the tortilla's edges inward and roll it up.

8. Continue with the leftover tortillas.

9. Enjoy a tasty, high-protein meal by serving the Sweet Potato and Black Bean meal Burrito right away.

- *Lunch: Grilled Chicken Salad with Mixed Greens*

Ingredients:

- 2 boneless, skinless chicken breasts
- 6 cups mixed salad greens (such as lettuce, spinach, arugula)
- 1 cup cherry tomatoes, halved
- 1/2 cucumber, sliced

- 1/4 red onion, thinly sliced
- 1/4 cup crumbled feta cheese
- 1/4 cup sliced almonds
- Salt and pepper to taste
- Olive oil for grilling

For the Marinade:

- 2 tablespoons olive oil
- 2 cloves garlic, minced
- 1 teaspoon dried oregano
- 1 teaspoon dried thyme
- Juice of 1 lemon
- Salt and pepper to taste

For the Dressing:

- 3 tablespoons extra virgin olive oil
- 2 tablespoons balsamic vinegar
- 1 teaspoon Dijon mustard
- 1 teaspoon honey
- Salt and pepper to taste

Instructions:

1. Combine the marinade ingredients in a small bowl, whisking in the lemon juice, olive oil, minced garlic, dried oregano, dried thyme, salt, and pepper.

2. Transfer the chicken breasts to a shallow dish or plastic bag that can be sealed, and cover them with the marinade. Make sure the chicken has a good coating. Refrigerate for a minimum of 30 minutes or for up to 4 hours after covering or sealing.

3. Set the grill's temperature to medium-high. To keep the grill grates from sticking, lightly grease them with olive oil.

4. Take out the marinated chicken breasts and throw away any extra marinade. Add salt and pepper to the chicken to season it.

5. Place the chicken breasts on the grill and cook for 6 to 8 minutes on each side, or until the internal temperature reaches 165°F (75°C). Before slicing, take them from the grill and give them some time to rest.

6. Prepare the salad ingredients while the chicken is roasting. Combine the mixed salad greens, sliced almonds, cucumber, red onion, crumbled feta cheese, and cherry tomatoes in a big bowl.

7. Combine the extra virgin olive oil, balsamic vinegar, Dijon mustard, honey, salt, and pepper in a small bowl to make the dressing.

8. After the chicken has rested, finely slice it.

9. Distribute the mixed greens and additional ingredients among serving dishes to make the salad. Add some grilled chicken pieces on the top of each salad.

10. Cover the salads with a drizzle of balsamic vinaigrette dressing.

11. Present the grilled chicken salad right away with mixed greens, and dig in!

- Dinner: Baked Cod with Lemon-Dill Sauce, Quinoa, and Roasted Vegetables

Baked Cod with Lemon-Dill Sauce:

Ingredients:

- 4 cod filets (about 6 ounces each)
- Salt and pepper to taste
- 2 tablespoons olive oil
- 2 tablespoons fresh lemon juice
- 2 cloves garlic, minced
- 1 tablespoon chopped fresh dill
- Lemon wedges for serving

Instructions:

1. Set the oven temperature to 400°F, or 200°C.
2. Arrange the cod filets on a parchment paper-lined baking sheet.
3. Use salt and pepper to season the cod filets.

4. Combine the olive oil, lemon juice, minced garlic, and chopped fresh dill in a small bowl.

5. Cover the cod filets with a drizzle of the lemon-dill sauce.

6. Bake the fish for 12 to 15 minutes in a preheated oven, or until it is opaque and flakes readily with a fork.

7. Take the baked cod with lemon-dill sauce out of the oven and serve it with lemon wedges on the side.

Quinoa:

Ingredients:

- 1 cup quinoa, rinsed
- 2 cups water or vegetable broth
- Salt to taste
- Optional: chopped fresh parsley or cilantro for garnish

Instructions:

1. Place the quinoa and the vegetable broth or water in a medium pot.

2. Place over medium-high heat and bring to a boil.

3. Simmer the quinoa for 15 to 20 minutes, covered, or until the liquid is absorbed, on low heat.

4. Using a fork, fluff the quinoa and add salt to taste.

5. If preferred, garnish with finely chopped fresh cilantro or parsley.

Roasted Vegetables:

Ingredients:

- Assorted vegetables (such as bell peppers, zucchini, cherry tomatoes, red onion, etc.), chopped
- 2 tablespoons olive oil
- Salt and pepper to taste
- Optional: dried herbs (such as thyme, rosemary, or oregano)

Instructions:

1. Set the oven temperature to 400°F, or 200°C.

2. Arrange the chopped veggies on a parchment paper-lined baking pan.

3. Add a drizzle of olive oil and season with the optional dried herbs, salt, and pepper.

4. Toss the veggies in the oil and seasonings to ensure they are equally coated.

5. Roast the veggies for 20 to 25 minutes in a preheated oven, or until they are soft and have begun to caramelize.

- *Snack: Mixed Nuts and Seeds Trail Mix*

Ingredients:

- 1 cup almonds
- 1 cup cashews
- 1 cup walnuts
- 1/2 cup pumpkin seeds (pepitas)
- 1/2 cup sunflower seeds
- 1/4 cup dried cranberries
- 1/4 cup raisins
- 1/4 cup dried apricots, chopped
- 1/4 cup dark chocolate chips (optional)
- 1 teaspoon cinnamon (optional)
- 1/2 teaspoon sea salt (optional)

Instructions:

1. Place the almonds, cashews, walnuts, pumpkin seeds, and sunflower seeds in a large mixing basin.
2. Fill the bowl with the chopped dried apricots, raisins, dried cranberries, and dark chocolate chips (if using).
3. For added taste, you may top the mixture with sea salt and cinnamon, if you'd like.
4. Combine everything and toss until thoroughly mixed.

5. To make it simple to munch on the move, transfer the mixed nuts and seeds trail mix to an airtight container or separate it into individual, portion-sized bags.
6. Trail mix can be kept for up to two weeks in a cool, dry location.

You may alter this recipe for trail mix by substituting your preferred dried fruits, nuts, or seeds for any of the ingredients. For variation, you may also add other items like dried pineapple, pretzel bits, or coconut flakes.

Day 2:

- Breakfast: Chia Seed Pudding with Fresh Mango

Ingredients:

- 1/4 cup chia seeds
- 1 cup milk (dairy or non-dairy)
- 1 tablespoon honey or maple syrup (optional, for sweetness)

- 1/2 teaspoon vanilla extract
- 1 ripe mango, peeled and diced
- Optional toppings: sliced almonds, shredded coconut, fresh berries

Instructions:

1. Place the milk, chia seeds, vanilla extract, honey (if using), and maple syrup in a jar or mixing dish. Mix well to blend.
2. To help the chia seeds thicken and absorb the liquid, cover the dish or jar and refrigerate for at least two hours, but preferably overnight.
3. Give the chia seed pudding a thorough stir to break up any clumps after it has thickened to the consistency you wish.
4. Transfer the chia seed pudding into jars or serving dishes when it's time to serve.
5. Add diced fresh mango on the top of each dish.
6. Optional: For added taste and texture, garnish with fresh berries, shredded coconut, or almond slices.
7. Present the Chia Seed Pudding with Fresh Mango right away, then savor it!

- Lunch: Lentil and Vegetable Curry with Brown Rice

Ingredients:

- 1 cup brown lentils, rinsed and drained
- 2 cups vegetable broth or water
- 1 tablespoon olive oil or coconut oil
- 1 onion, diced
- 3 cloves garlic, minced
- 1 tablespoon grated ginger
- 1 tablespoon curry powder
- 1 teaspoon ground cumin
- 1 teaspoon ground turmeric
- 1/2 teaspoon ground coriander
- 1/4 teaspoon cayenne pepper (optional, for added heat)
- 1 can (14 oz) diced tomatoes
- 1 can (14 oz) coconut milk
- 2 cups mixed vegetables (such as bell peppers, carrots, zucchini, cauliflower, etc.), chopped
- Salt and pepper to taste
- Cooked brown rice for serving
- Fresh cilantro leaves for garnish

Instructions:

1. Heat the olive oil in a big saucepan or Dutch oven over medium heat.
2. Cook the chopped onion in the saucepan for about five minutes, or until it becomes tender.

3. Add the grated ginger and minced garlic, and simmer for a further one to two minutes, or until fragrant.

4. Fill the saucepan with curry powder, ground cumin, ground turmeric, ground coriander, and, if desired, cayenne pepper. After giving the onions and spices a quick stir, simmer for a minute.

5. Add the chopped tomatoes and coconut milk, stirring to mix in the juices.

6. Pour the water or vegetable broth into the saucepan and add the washed and drained brown lentils.

7. Once the curry reaches a boil, lower the heat to a simmer and let it uncovered for twenty to twenty-five minutes, or until the lentils are soft and the sauce has thickened.

8. Once the veggies are cooked to your preference, stir in the chopped mixed vegetables and simmer for a further 10 to 15 minutes.

9. Add salt and pepper to taste when preparing the lentil and vegetable curry.

10. Spoon hot curry over brown rice that has been prepared.

11. Before serving, garnish with fresh cilantro leaves.

- Dinner: Mushroom and Spinach Frittata, Sweet Potato and Kale Hash

Mushroom and Spinach Frittata:

Ingredients:
- 8 large eggs
- 1/4 cup milk (dairy or non-dairy)
- Salt and pepper to taste
- 1 tablespoon olive oil
- 1 small onion, diced
- 8 ounces mushrooms, sliced
- 2 cups fresh spinach leaves
- 1/4 cup grated Parmesan cheese (optional)
- Fresh herbs for garnish (such as parsley or chives)

Instructions:

1. Set the oven temperature to 175°C, or 350°F.
2. Combine the eggs, milk, salt, and pepper in a large mixing basin and whisk until thoroughly blended. Put aside.
3. In a large ovenproof skillet, heat the olive oil over medium heat.
4. Fill the skillet with sliced mushrooms and chopped onion. Cook until the onions are tender and the mushrooms are golden brown, stirring from time to time.

5. Cook the fresh spinach leaves in the pan for a further one to two minutes, or until they have wilted.

6. Evenly divide the veggies in the skillet by pouring the egg mixture over them.

7. Cook the frittata for two to three minutes without stirring, or until the edges begin to firm.

8. Evenly distribute grated Parmesan cheese, if using, on top of the frittata.

9. Place the pan in the oven and bake for 15 to 20 minutes, or until the top of the frittata is gently browned.

10. Take the frittata out of the oven and allow it to cool slightly before slicing.

11. Before serving, garnish with fresh herbs.

Sweet Potato and Kale Hash:

Ingredients:

- 2 medium sweet potatoes, peeled and diced
- 1 tablespoon olive oil
- 1 small onion, diced
- 2 cloves garlic, minced
- 2 cups chopped kale leaves
- Salt and pepper to taste
- **Optional toppings**: fried or poached eggs, avocado slices, hot sauce

Instructions:

1. In a big skillet over medium heat, warm up the olive oil.

2. Add the diced sweet potatoes to the skillet and simmer for 8 to 10 minutes, turning often, or until they are soft and lightly browned.

3. When the onion is transparent and aromatic, add the chopped onion and minced garlic to the skillet and simmer for an additional two to three minutes.

4. Add the chopped kale leaves and simmer for two to three minutes, or until they are soft and wilted.

5. Add salt and pepper to taste when adding the sweet potato and kale combination.

6. Present the heated Sweet Potato and Kale Hash with the option of adding extras like avocado slices, spicy sauce, or fried or poached eggs.

- Snack: Sliced Apple with Almond Butter

Ingredients:

- 1 apple (any variety you prefer)
- 2 tablespoons almond butter (or any nut or seed butter of your choice)

- Optional toppings: cinnamon, honey, chopped nuts, shredded coconut, or dried fruit

Instructions:

1. Give the apple a good wash and dry.
2. After cutting off the seeds and core, thinly slice the apple into rounds or wedges.
3. Drizzle a thick layer of almond butter over each apple slice.
4. Optional: Top the almond butter with chopped nuts, shredded coconut, dried fruit, or any other desired garnish. You may also drizzle honey over it or sprinkle cinnamon on top.
5. Put the apple slices in a platter or dish arrangement.
6. Present right away and have your tasty and wholesome snack!

Day 3:

- *Breakfast: Whole Grain Pancakes with Fresh Berries*

Ingredients:

- 1 cup whole wheat flour
- 1/2 cup oat flour (you can make your own by blending oats in a food processor until fine)
- 2 tablespoons ground flaxseed (optional, for added fiber and omega-3 fatty acids)
- 1 tablespoon baking powder
- 1/4 teaspoon salt
- 1 cup milk (dairy or non-dairy)
- 1 egg
- 2 tablespoons honey or maple syrup
- 2 tablespoons melted butter or coconut oil
- Fresh berries (such as strawberries, blueberries, raspberries, etc.) for topping
- Maple syrup or honey for serving

Instructions:

1. Combine the whole wheat flour, oat flour, baking powder, powdered flaxseed (if using), and salt in a large mixing basin.
2. Whisk the egg, milk, melted butter or coconut oil, honey or maple syrup, and other ingredients in another bowl.
3. Add the wet mixture to the dry mixture and whisk just until blended. Take care not to overmix; a little lumpiness in the batter is OK.

4. Turn up the heat to medium on a nonstick skillet or griddle. Apply a thin layer of butter or oil on the surface.

5. For each pancake, add around 1/4 cup of batter to the skillet.

6. Cook the pancakes for two to three minutes, or until the edges seem firm and bubbles appear on the surface.

7. After flipping the pancakes, heat for a further one to two minutes, or until they are cooked through and golden brown.

8. Continue with the leftover batter, lubricating the skillet as necessary.

9. Present the Whole Grain Pancakes with a dollop of honey or maple syrup and fresh berries on top.

- Lunch: Caprese Quinoa Bowl

Ingredients:

- 1 cup quinoa, rinsed
- 2 cups water or vegetable broth
- 2 cups cherry tomatoes, halved
- 1 cup fresh mozzarella balls (bocconcini), halved
- 1/4 cup fresh basil leaves, chopped
- 2 tablespoons extra virgin olive oil

- 1 tablespoon balsamic vinegar
- Salt and pepper to taste
- Balsamic glaze for drizzling (optional)

Instructions:

1. Put the quinoa and the vegetable broth or water in a saucepan. After bringing to a boil, lower the heat to a simmer, cover, and cook the quinoa for 15 to 20 minutes, or until it is tender and the liquid has been absorbed. Using a fork, fluff the quinoa and let it cool somewhat.

2. Place the cooked quinoa, chopped fresh basil leaves, half cherry tomatoes, and halved fresh mozzarella balls in a large mixing bowl.

3. To create the dressing, combine the extra virgin olive oil and balsamic vinegar in a small bowl.

4. Drizzle the quinoa mixture with the dressing, tossing to cover everything thoroughly.

5. Use salt and pepper to taste while preparing the Caprese quinoa bowl.

6. Distribute the combination of quinoa among serving dishes.

7. **Optional:** For added taste, drizzle balsamic glaze over the top of each bowl.

8. Present the Caprese Quinoa Bowls right away and savor them!

- Dinner: Teriyaki Turkey Stir-Fry with Quinoa

Ingredients:

- 1 cup quinoa, rinsed
- 2 cups water or chicken broth
- 1 tablespoon olive oil
- 1 pound turkey breast, thinly sliced
- 2 cups mixed vegetables (such as bell peppers, broccoli, carrots, snap peas, etc.), sliced
- 3 cloves garlic, minced
- 1/4 cup teriyaki sauce
- 2 tablespoons soy sauce (or tamari for gluten-free option)
- 1 tablespoon honey or brown sugar
- 1 teaspoon sesame oil
- 1 tablespoon cornstarch mixed with 2 tablespoons water (optional, for thickening the sauce)
- Sesame seeds and chopped green onions for garnish

Instructions:

1. Place the washed quinoa and chicken broth or water in a saucepan. After bringing to a boil, lower the heat to a simmer, cover, and cook the quinoa for

15 to 20 minutes, or until it is tender and the liquid has been absorbed. Using a fork, fluff and set aside.

2. Heat the olive oil in a big pan or wok over medium-high heat.

3. When the turkey breast is cooked through and no longer pink, add it to the skillet with the slices and stir-fry it for three to four minutes. Take out and place aside from the skillet.

4. Add the chopped garlic and mixed veggies to the same skillet. Stir-fry the veggies for 4–5 minutes, or until they are crisp-tender.

5. Add the cooked turkey and veggies back to the skillet.

6. Combine the soy sauce, honey (or brown sugar), sesame oil, and teriyaki sauce in a small bowl. Over the turkey and veggies in the pan, pour the sauce.

7. To thicken the sauce, if preferred, add the cornstarch-water combination to the skillet. Mix well to blend.

8. Cook for a further one to two minutes, or until the sauce has cooked through and thickened.

9. Top cooked quinoa with Teriyaki Turkey Stir-Fry.

10. Before serving, garnish with chopped green onions and sesame seeds.

- Snack: Greek Yogurt and Berry Parfait

Ingredients:

- 1 cup Greek yogurt or dairy-free yogurt
- 1 cup mixed berries (such as strawberries, blueberries, raspberries, and blackberries), fresh or frozen
- 1 tablespoon honey or maple syrup (optional, for added sweetness)
- 1/4 cup granola
- Fresh mint leaves for garnish (optional)

Instructions:

1. Thaw frozen berries in the fridge or at room temperature until they become somewhat softer, if using frozen berries.
2. Gently stir the Greek yogurt and maple syrup (if using) in a small bowl until thoroughly blended.
3. Layer the Greek yogurt mixture, mixed berries, and granola into serving glasses or jars. Continue layering until the glasses are full.
4. Line the bottom of each glass with a layer of Greek yogurt, then add a layer of mixed berries, and finally top with granola. Until you reach the top of the glass, keep adding layers.
5. If preferred, add some more berries and fresh mint leaves to the top of each parfait.

6. You can either serve the Greek yogurt and berry parfait right away or put it in the fridge to serve later.

Day 4:

- Breakfast: Berry Bliss Smoothie

Ingredients:

- 1 cup mixed berries (such as strawberries, blueberries, raspberries, and blackberries), fresh or frozen
- 1 ripe banana
- 1/2 cup Greek yogurt or dairy-free yogurt
- 1/2 cup almond milk or any milk of your choice
- 1 tablespoon honey or maple syrup (optional, for added sweetness)
- 1 tablespoon chia seeds or flaxseeds (optional, for added fiber and omega-3 fatty acids)
- Ice cubes (if using fresh berries)

Instructions:

1. To cool the smoothie, add a few ice cubes to the blender if you're using fresh berries.

2. Fill the blender with the mixed berries, ripe banana, Greek yogurt, almond milk, honey, maple syrup, or flaxseeds, if desired.

3. Blend until creamy and smooth, stopping the blender occasionally to scrape down the sides to make sure all the ingredients are completely mixed.

4. After tasting the smoothie, taste it again and add additional honey or almond milk if needed to modify the sweetness or thickness.

5. Pour the smoothie into glasses and serve right away when it achieves the consistency you've desired.

- *Lunch: Turkey and Avocado Lettuce Wraps*

Ingredients:

- 1 lb ground turkey (or cooked turkey breast, shredded)
- 1 avocado, diced
- 1/2 red bell pepper, diced
- 1/4 red onion, finely chopped
- 1/4 cup fresh cilantro, chopped
- Juice of 1 lime

- Salt and pepper to taste
- Lettuce leaves (such as butter lettuce, romaine, or iceberg) for wrapping
- **Optional toppings**: diced tomatoes, shredded cheese, salsa, sour cream

Instructions:

1. In a skillet over medium heat, brown and fully cook the ground turkey, if using. Empty any extra fat. Use your hands or forks to shred the cooked turkey breast.
2. Add the diced avocado, diced red bell pepper, finely sliced red onion, chopped cilantro, and cooked turkey (or shredded turkey breast) to a large mixing bowl.
3. Drizzle with the lime juice and stir everything together.
4. Add salt and pepper to taste when spicing the turkey and avocado combination.
5. Using individual lettuce leaves as wraps, spoon the turkey and avocado mixture onto them.
6. **Optional**: Top the turkey mixture with extras like sour cream, salsa, shredded cheese, or sliced tomatoes.
7. Using toothpicks if necessary, roll up the lettuce leaves to enclose the filling.
8. Present Turkey and Avocado Lettuce Wraps right away, and savor them as a nutritious and light meal!

Spaghetti Squash with Tomato Basil Sauce:

Ingredients:

- 1 medium spaghetti squash
- 2 tablespoons olive oil
- Salt and pepper to taste
- 2 cups tomato basil sauce (homemade or store-bought)
- Grated Parmesan cheese for serving (optional)
- Fresh basil leaves for garnish

Instructions:

Set the oven temperature to 400°F, or 200°C.
2. Scoop out the seeds after cutting the spaghetti squash in half lengthwise.
3. Season with salt and pepper and drizzle olive oil over the sliced sides of the spaghetti squash halves.
4. Lay the spaghetti squash halves on a baking sheet covered with parchment paper, cut side down.

5. Roast the squash for 40 to 50 minutes in a preheated oven, or until it is fork-tender.

6. After allowing the spaghetti squash to cool slightly, scrape the flesh into "spaghetti-like" strands with a fork.

7. In a saucepan, reheat the tomato basil sauce over medium heat until it is well heated.

8. Present the baked spaghetti squash with a tomato basil sauce on top. If preferred, garnish with freshly chopped basil leaves and grated Parmesan cheese.

Grilled Chicken with Mango Avocado Salsa:

Ingredients:

- 2 boneless, skinless chicken breasts
- 1 tablespoon olive oil
- Salt and pepper to taste
- 1 ripe mango, peeled and diced
- 1 ripe avocado, peeled and diced
- 1/4 cup diced red onion
- 1/4 cup chopped fresh cilantro
- Juice of 1 lime
- Salt and pepper to taste

Instructions:

1. Turn the heat up to medium-high on your grill or grill pan.

2. Season the chicken breasts with salt and pepper after rubbing them with olive oil.

3. Cook the chicken breasts on the grill for 6 to 8 minutes on each side, or until they are cooked through and no longer have a pink core. Depending on the thickness of the chicken breasts, cooking times might change.

4. Make the mango-avocado salsa while the chicken grills. Diced mango, avocado, red onion, chopped fresh cilantro, lime juice, salt, and pepper should all be combined in a dish. Gently stir until thoroughly blended.

5. After the chicken is done, take it from the grill and let it rest for a few minutes to rest before slicing.

6. Present the grilled chicken with a mango-avocado salsa on top.

Savor this tasty and wholesome dinner of Grilled Chicken with Mango Avocado Salsa and Spaghetti Squash with Tomato Basil Sauce!

- Snack: Roasted Chickpeas Snack

Ingredients:

- 2 cans (15 oz each) chickpeas (garbanzo beans), drained and rinsed
- 2 tablespoons olive oil
- 1 teaspoon ground cumin
- 1 teaspoon smoked paprika
- 1/2 teaspoon garlic powder
- 1/2 teaspoon onion powder
- 1/4 teaspoon cayenne pepper (optional, for heat)
- Salt to taste

Instructions:

1. Set the oven temperature to 400°F, or 200°C. For easier cleanup, line a baking pan with aluminum foil or parchment paper.

2. After the chickpeas have been rinsed and drained, spread them out on a fresh kitchen towel and pat dry. Eliminate any fallen skin that becomes loose.

3. Toss the dry chickpeas with olive oil in a big mixing basin until they are well covered.

4. Combine the ground cumin, smoked paprika, onion and garlic powders, salt, and cayenne pepper (if using) in a small bowl.

5. Distribute the spice blend onto the chickpeas and stir until they are thoroughly coated.

6. Arrange the seasoned chickpeas on the baking sheet that has been prepared in a single layer.

7. Roast the chickpeas for 20 to 30 minutes in a preheated oven, stirring the pan halfway through, or until they are crispy and browned.

8. After roasting, take the chickpeas out of the oven and let them cool for a short while on the baking sheet.

9. To enjoy the roasted chickpeas later, serve them warm as a snack or let them cool fully before putting them in an airtight container.

Day 5:

- *Breakfast: Avocado Toast with Poached Egg*

Ingredients:

- 2 slices whole grain bread
- 1 ripe avocado
- 2 eggs
- Salt and pepper to taste
- Optional toppings: red pepper flakes, sliced cherry tomatoes, chopped fresh herbs (such as cilantro or parsley), crumbled feta cheese

Instructions:

1. Toast the whole grain bread slices until crispy and golden brown.

2. Prepare the avocado while the bread is toasting. Remove the pit from the avocado, cut it in half, and scoop out the flesh into a small dish. Using a fork, mash the avocado until it's smooth and creamy. To taste, add salt and pepper for seasoning.

3. Simmer the water gently in a medium pot. To aid in the coagulation of the egg whites, add a small amount of vinegar to the water.

4. Break one egg into a ramekin or little dish. Carefully push the egg into the middle of the gently swirling vortex in the heating water using a spoon. Continue with the other egg.

5. Poach the eggs for three to four minutes, or until the yolks are still runny but the whites are set.

6. Evenly distribute the mashed avocado over the slices of toasted bread while the eggs are poaching.

7. Take the poached eggs out of the water with a slotted spoon and discard any extra water. Every avocado toast should have one poached egg on top of it.

8. To taste, add salt and pepper to the poached eggs.

9. Optional garnishes for the avocado toast are crumbled feta cheese, chopped fresh herbs, sliced cherry tomatoes, and red pepper flakes.

10. Present the Avocado Toast with Poached Egg right away, then savor it!

- *Lunch: Chickpea and Vegetable Stir-Fry*

Ingredients:

- 1 can (15 oz) chickpeas, drained and rinsed
- 2 cups mixed vegetables (broccoli, bell peppers, snap peas, carrots, etc.), chopped
- 1 tablespoon sesame oil or vegetable oil
- 3 cloves garlic, minced
- 1 tablespoon ginger, grated
- 2 tablespoons soy sauce
- 1 tablespoon hoisin sauce
- 1 teaspoon rice vinegar
- 1 teaspoon sesame seeds (optional)
- Green onions, sliced for garnish (optional)
- Cooked brown rice or quinoa for serving

Instructions:

1. Heat the sesame oil in a big pan or wok over medium-high heat.
2. Sauté the grated ginger and chopped garlic in the heated oil for about 30 seconds, or until fragrant.

3. Stir-fry the mixed veggies in the skillet for three to five minutes, or until they start to get tender but still have a crisp texture.

4. Stir the veggies and the drained chickpeas together.

5. Combine rice vinegar, hoisin sauce, and soy sauce in a small bowl. After adding the sauce, toss to ensure that the veggies and chickpeas are uniformly coated.

6. Stir-fry the chickpeas for a further two to three minutes, or until they are well cooked.

7. Add sesame seeds to the stir-fry, if using, and toss to mix.

8. Spoon the Chickpea and Vegetable Stir-Fry over warm quinoa or brown rice.

9. You can choose to add sliced green onions as a garnish.

- Dinner: Cauliflower Fried Rice with Tofu

Ingredients:

- 1 head cauliflower, riced (or about 4 cups cauliflower rice)
- 1 tablespoon sesame oil
- 2 tablespoons soy sauce (or tamari for gluten-free option)

- 2 cloves garlic, minced
- 1 tablespoon grated ginger
- 1 block extra firm tofu, pressed and diced
- 1 cup mixed vegetables (such as carrots, peas, corn, and bell peppers)
- 2 green onions, sliced
- 2 eggs, beaten (optional)
- Salt and pepper to taste
- Sesame seeds and sliced green onions for garnish

Instructions:

1. In a food processor, pulse the cauliflower florets until they resemble rice grains to make the cauliflower rice. You may also use prepackaged cauliflower rice.

2. Heat the sesame oil in a big skillet or wok over medium heat.

3. Add the grated ginger and minced garlic to the skillet and cook for one to two minutes, or until fragrant.

4. Add the diced tofu to the skillet and heat, turning periodically, until the tofu is gently browned, about 5 to 7 minutes.

5. Transfer the mixed veggies to one side of the pan and push the tofu to the other. Simmer the veggies for 3–4 minutes, or until they are soft.

6. Push the veggies and tofu to one side of the skillet and fill the empty space with the beaten eggs.

After the eggs are fully cooked, stir them into the tofu and veggies.

7. Add the cauliflower rice to the skillet along with the eggs, veggies, and tofu, and mix to incorporate.

8. To ensure that everything is properly coated, drizzle soy sauce (or tamari) over the cauliflower rice mixture and toss.

9. Cook the cauliflower rice for five to seven minutes, stirring now and again, until it's soft and well cooked.

10. Add pepper and salt to taste.

11. **Optional**: Before serving, garnish with sliced green onions and sesame seeds.

- Snack: Cucumber and Hummus Bites

Ingredients:

- 1 large cucumber
- Hummus (store-bought or homemade)
- Cherry tomatoes, sliced (optional)
- Black olives, sliced (optional)
- Fresh parsley or dill for garnish (optional)

Instructions:

1. Give the cucumber a good wash and use paper towels to pat dry.

2. Cut the cucumber into rounds that are around half an inch thick.

3. To make a little well for the hummus, you can, if you'd like, use a miniature spoon or melon baller to scoop out a small depression in the middle of each cucumber slice.

4. Place a little dollop of hummus onto every slice of cucumber.

5. **Optional:** For extra taste and appearance, top each cucumber and hummus bite with a cherry tomato slice, a black olive slice, or a sprig of fresh parsley or dill.

6. Transfer the cucumber and hummus morsels to a dish for presentation.

7. Serve right away as a wholesome and revitalizing snack or appetizer.

Day 6:

- Breakfast: Quinoa Breakfast Bowl

Ingredients:

- 1/2 cup quinoa, rinsed
- 1 cup water or milk (dairy or non-dairy)
- 1 tablespoon honey or maple syrup (optional)
- 1/2 teaspoon ground cinnamon
- 1/4 teaspoon vanilla extract
- Pinch of salt
- Fresh fruit (such as berries, sliced bananas, diced mango, etc.)
- Nuts or seeds (such as almonds, walnuts, chia seeds, pumpkin seeds, etc.)
- Greek yogurt or coconut yogurt (optional)
- Honey or maple syrup for drizzling (optional)

Instructions:

1. Place the washed quinoa and milk or water in a small pot. Heat to a boil on a medium setting.
2. Simmer the quinoa for 15 to 20 minutes, covered, or until the liquid is absorbed, on low heat.
3. After the quinoa is cooked, take it off the stove and cover it for five minutes.
4. Using a fork, fluff the quinoa and mix in the ground cinnamon, vanilla essence, honey or maple syrup (if using), and a little amount of salt.
5. Spoon cooked quinoa into dishes for dishing.
6. Add fresh fruit, nuts, or seeds, and, if like, a dollop of Greek or coconut yogurt to the top of each bowl.

7. If preferred, drizzle with more honey or maple syrup for added sweetness.
8. Present your wholesome and filling Quinoa Breakfast Bowl right away and savor it!

Feel free to add your preferred flavorings and toppings to your Quinoa Breakfast Bowl. Additionally, you may prepare a bigger quantity of quinoa in advance and keep it refrigerated for simple and quick breakfasts all week long.

- *Lunch: Tomato and Basil Avocado Toast*

Ingredients:

- 2 slices whole grain bread
- 1 ripe avocado
- 1 medium tomato, sliced
- Fresh basil leaves
- Salt and pepper to taste
- Red pepper flakes (optional, for added spice)
- Lemon juice (optional, for extra flavor)

Instructions:

1. Toast the whole grain bread slices until crispy and golden brown.

2. Use a fork to mash the ripe avocado in a small bowl while the bread is toasting. If preferred, add a squeeze of lemon juice and season with salt and pepper.

3. After the bread is done, equally distribute the mashed avocado over each piece.

4. Place some fresh tomato slices on top of the avocado toast.

5. Tear a few leaves of fresh basil and distribute them on top of the tomato slices.

6. For an extra fiery burst, feel free to top with red pepper flakes.

7. Present the Tomato and Basil Avocado Toast right away, and savor it as a wholesome and delectable alternative for breakfast, brunch, or a snack!

- Dinner: Baked Chicken Breast with Roasted Vegetables, Cauliflower Crust Margherita Pizza

Baked Chicken Breast with Roasted Vegetables:

Ingredients:

- 2 boneless, skinless chicken breasts
- 2 tablespoons olive oil
- 2 cloves garlic, minced
- 1 teaspoon dried Italian seasoning
- Salt and pepper to taste
- Assorted vegetables (such as bell peppers, zucchini, cherry tomatoes, red onion, etc.), chopped
- Fresh herbs for garnish (such as parsley or basil)

Instructions:

1. Set the oven temperature to 400°F, or 200°C.
2. Spread some olive oil on the chicken breasts and put them in a baking tray.
3. Give the chicken breasts a rubdown with minced garlic and dry Italian spice. Add pepper and salt for seasoning.
4. In the baking dish, arrange the chopped veggies around the chicken breasts.
5. Roast for 20 to 25 minutes, or until the chicken is well cooked and the veggies are soft, in a preheated oven.
6. Take the chicken out of the oven and let it sit for a few minutes before slicing.
7. Before serving, garnish with fresh herbs.

Cauliflower Crust Margherita Pizza:

Ingredients:

- 1 medium head cauliflower, riced
- 1 egg
- 1/2 cup shredded mozzarella cheese
- 1/4 cup grated Parmesan cheese
- 1 teaspoon dried Italian seasoning
- Salt and pepper to taste
- 1/2 cup marinara sauce
- Fresh basil leaves
- Sliced tomatoes
- Fresh mozzarella cheese, sliced

Instructions:

1. Set the oven's temperature to 425°F (220°C).
2. Put the riced cauliflower in a bowl that is safe to microwave and heat it for five to six minutes, or until it becomes tender.
3. After allowing the cauliflower to cool slightly, place it on a fresh kitchen towel and wring out any extra liquid.
4. Place the cauliflower, egg, grated Parmesan cheese, dry Italian seasoning, shredded mozzarella cheese, and salt and pepper in a mixing bowl. Mix until well blended.

5. Press the cauliflower mixture into the shape of a thin crust by lining a baking sheet with parchment paper.
6. Bake the cauliflower crust for 15 to 20 minutes, or until it is firm and golden brown, in a preheated oven.
7. Take the cauliflower crust out of the oven and cover it with marinara sauce.
8. Add sliced tomatoes, fresh basil leaves, and slices of mozzarella cheese on top.
9. Put the pizza back in the oven and bake it for a further five to seven minutes, or until the cheese is bubbling and melted.
10. Cut the Cauliflower Crust Margherita Pizza into pieces and serve it with the Roasted Vegetables and Baked Chicken Breast.

- Snack: Walnut and Grape Bruschetta

Ingredients:

- 1 French baguette, sliced into 1/2-inch thick rounds
- 1 cup red seedless grapes, halved
- 1/2 cup walnuts, chopped
- 4 ounces goat cheese

- Honey, for drizzling
- Fresh thyme leaves, for garnish
- Olive oil, for drizzling
- Salt and pepper to taste

Instructions:

1. Set the oven temperature to 375°F, or 190°C.
2. Arrange the baguette slices on an oven tray and gently mist them with olive oil. Add a dash of pepper and salt for seasoning.
3. Toast the baguette slices for 8 to 10 minutes, or until they are crisp and gently brown.
4. Combine the chopped walnuts and the half-grapes in a small bowl.
5. Top each piece of toasted bread with a heaping tablespoon of goat cheese.
6. Place a layer of the grape and walnut mixture on top of each baguette slice, carefully pressing it in place.
7. For a hint of sweetness, drizzle honey over the top of each bruschetta.
8. Add some fresh thyme leaves to the walnut and grape bruschetta as a garnish.
9. Serve as a snack or appetizer right away.

Day 7:

- Breakfast: Smoked Salmon and Cream Cheese Bagel

Ingredients:

- 1 whole grain bagel, sliced and toasted
- Light cream cheese
- Smoked salmon
- Sliced cucumber and tomato

Instructions:

1. Toast the whole grain bagel until it reaches the crispiness you like.
2. Top each half of the toasted bagel with a layer of light cream cheese.
3. Place smoked salmon slices over the cream cheese.
4. To add freshness and crunch to the smoked salmon, thinly slice a tomato and cucumber over it.
5. For extra taste, you may optionally add a squeeze of lemon juice or a sprinkling of fresh dill.
6. To make a sandwich, place the second half of the bagel on top.

7. Present the Bagel with Smoked Salmon and Cream Cheese right away, and enjoy a delicious and heart-healthy brunch or breakfast.

- Lunch: Vegetable and Quinoa Stuffed Bell Peppers

Ingredients:

- 4 large bell peppers, any color
- 1 cup quinoa, rinsed
- 2 cups vegetable broth or water
- 1 tablespoon olive oil
- 1 small onion, diced
- 2 cloves garlic, minced
- 1 carrot, diced
- 1 zucchini, diced
- 1 cup cherry tomatoes, halved
- 1 cup cooked black beans (or canned, rinsed and drained)
- 1 teaspoon ground cumin
- 1 teaspoon smoked paprika
- Salt and pepper to taste
- 1/4 cup chopped fresh parsley or cilantro
- 1/2 cup shredded cheese (such as cheddar, mozzarella, or pepper jack), optional

Instructions:

1. Set the oven temperature to 375°F, or 190°C.
2. Slice off the bell peppers' tops, then take out the seeds and membranes. Put aside.
3. Place the quinoa and water or vegetable broth in a medium pot. After bringing to a boil, lower the heat to a simmer, cover, and cook the quinoa for 15 to 20 minutes, or until it is tender and the liquid has been absorbed.
4. Heat the olive oil in a big pan over medium heat. Add the chopped onion and garlic, and simmer for 3–4 minutes, or until softened.
5. Cook the chopped zucchini and carrot in the pan for a further four to five minutes, or until the veggies are soft.
6. Add the cooked black beans and cherry tomatoes cut in half and cook for 2 to 3 minutes, or until well cooked.
7. Add salt, pepper, smoked paprika, and ground cumin to the vegetable mixture and toss to incorporate.
8. Include the cooked quinoa in the skillet along with the veggies, and thoroughly stir to include all the ingredients. Take off the heat.
9. Add finely chopped cilantro or parsley.
10. Add half of the shredded cheese, if using, to the quinoa and veggie combination.

11. Evenly distribute the quinoa and veggie mixture among the hollowed-out bell peppers using a spoon.

12. With the bell peppers packed, place them upright in a baking dish.

13. Optional: Top the filled bell peppers with the leftover shredded cheese.

14. Bake the baking dish for 25 to 30 minutes in a preheated oven covered with aluminum foil.

15. Take off the foil and continue baking for a further five to ten minutes, or until the cheese is bubbling and melted and the bell peppers are soft.

16. Before serving, take the cooked filled bell peppers out of the oven and allow them to cool for a few minutes.

- Dinner: Stuffed Zucchini Boats with Ground Turkey, Zesty Shrimp and Quinoa Salad

Ingredients:

For the Stuffed Zucchini Boats:

- 4 medium zucchinis
- 1 tablespoon olive oil
- 1/2 onion, diced

- 2 cloves garlic, minced
- 1/2 pound ground turkey
- 1 teaspoon Italian seasoning
- Salt and pepper to taste
- 1/2 cup marinara sauce
- 1/2 cup shredded mozzarella cheese
- Fresh basil leaves for garnish

For the Zesty Shrimp and Quinoa Salad:

- 1 cup quinoa, rinsed
- 1 1/2 cups water or chicken broth
- 1 pound shrimp, peeled and deveined
- 1 tablespoon olive oil
- 1 teaspoon paprika
- 1 teaspoon garlic powder
- 1/2 teaspoon chili powder
- Juice of 1 lemon
- Salt and pepper to taste
- 1/4 cup chopped fresh parsley
- 1/4 cup chopped red bell pepper
- 1/4 cup chopped cucumber
- 1/4 cup chopped cherry tomatoes
- 1/4 cup crumbled feta cheese (optional)
- Lemon wedges for serving

Instructions:

For the Stuffed Zucchini Boats:

1. Set the oven temperature to 375°F, or 190°C. Spread some olive oil on a baking dish.

2. Hollow out a "boat" by cutting each zucchini in half lengthwise and scooping out the seeds. After the baking dish is ready, put the zucchini boats inside.

3. Heat the olive oil in a pan over medium heat. Cook the minced garlic and chopped onion until they are tender.

4. Add the ground turkey to the skillet and heat, breaking it up with a spoon as it cooks, until it is browned.

5. Add salt, pepper, and Italian seasoning to the turkey mixture.

6. Drizzle each zucchini boat with marinara sauce. Spoon the cooked turkey mixture into each boat.

7. Cover the top of each filled zucchini boat with shredded mozzarella.

8. Bake the baking dish in the preheated oven for 20 to 25 minutes, or until the cheese is bubbling and melted and the zucchini is soft. Cover with foil.

9. Before serving, garnish with fresh basil leaves.

For the Zesty Shrimp and Quinoa Salad:

1. Water or chicken broth should be brought to a boil in a medium saucepan. Add the quinoa, cover, lower the heat to a simmer, and cook for 15 to 20

minutes, or until the quinoa is tender and the liquid has been absorbed. Using a fork, fluff, then allow to cool somewhat.

2. Thoroughly cover the shrimp with a mixture of olive oil, paprika, garlic powder, chili powder, lemon juice, salt, and pepper in a big bowl.

3. Turn up the heat to medium-high in a pan. Add the seasoned shrimp and cook, stirring, for 2 to 3 minutes on each side, or until opaque and pink. Take off from the heat and allow it to cool somewhat.

4. Add the chopped parsley, red bell pepper, cucumber, cherry tomatoes, and crumbled feta cheese (if using) to the bowl containing the cooked quinoa. Mix until well blended.

5. Spoon the quinoa salad and shrimp mixture onto serving dishes.

6. Present the Stuffed Zucchini Boats with Lemon Zesty Shrimp and Quinoa Salad, topped with slices of lemon.

- Snack: Dark Chocolate-Dipped Strawberries

Ingredients:

- Fresh strawberries, washed and dried
- Dark chocolate chips or chopped dark chocolate (at least 70% cocoa)
- **Optional toppings:** chopped nuts, shredded coconut, sprinkles, sea salt flakes, etc.

Instructions:

1. Use wax or parchment paper to line a baking pan.
2. Melt the chopped dark chocolate or dark chocolate chips in a heatproof dish over a double boiler or in the microwave for 30-second bursts, stirring until smooth.

Grasping each strawberry by its stem, submerge it into the liquefied chocolate, rotating it to cover approximately two-thirds of the fruit.

4. After letting any extra chocolate drip off, put the strawberry that has been dipped onto the baking sheet that has been ready.
5. While the chocolate is still wet, sprinkle your preferred toppings over the strawberries that have been dipped.
6. Use the remaining strawberries to repeat the dipping procedure.
7. Refrigerate the baking sheet for fifteen to twenty minutes, or until the chocolate sets.
8. After the dark chocolate-dipped strawberries have hardened, move them to a dish or plate.
9. Serve right away as a tasty treat or dessert.

CONCLUSION

We are happy that you have started your journey towards a healthy heart by looking through the **"Coronary Artery Disease Diet Cookbook for Newly Diagnosed."** You've started a journey that goes beyond simply altering your diet to include adopting a heart-healthy lifestyle that may significantly improve your general health.

We've worked hard to bring you easy and tasty meals in this cookbook that will please your palate as well as your body. We recognize that starting a new diet can be intimidating, particularly in light of a recent diagnosis. For this reason, we have concentrated on developing recipes that are simple to make and call for readily available ingredients that you can get at your neighborhood supermarket.

Our aim has been to make heart-healthy eating concepts approachable and clear to anyone, irrespective of food choices or level of culinary skill. We hope these pages will provide you with inspiration and direction to aid you on your path to better heart health, regardless of your level of experience in the kitchen.

The value of balance is one of the main ideas we've stressed throughout this cookbook. Finding the ideal nutrient balance to promote your heart health without sacrificing the foods you love is the goal of a heart-healthy diet, not deprivation or restriction. This entails consuming fewer saturated and trans fats, cholesterol, salt, whole grains, lean proteins, and added sweets while increasing your intake of fruits, vegetables, whole grains, lean meats, and healthy fats.

You may provide your body with the vitamins, minerals, antioxidants, and fiber it requires to flourish by putting an emphasis on complete, nutrient-dense meals. You'll discover that these meals are not only gratifying and tasty, but also heart-healthy. You have a variety of culinary options to explore on your heart-healthy path, from colorful salads and filling soups to tasty main courses and healthful snacks.

We've also urged you to think about other elements of a heart-healthy lifestyle, such as consistent physical activity, stress reduction, enough sleep, and social support, in addition to the food on your plate. We strongly advise you to look into ways to include these lifestyle aspects into your daily routine as they are essential for maintaining your general well-being and heart health.

As you go on your path to improved heart health, keep in mind that development is not always straight-line. It's acceptable if there are difficulties along the route. It's crucial that you remain dedicated to changing your life for the better, little by little. Honor your accomplishments, draw lessons from your failures, and never forget that every decision you make toward health is a positive step in the right path.

Lastly, we would like to send our warmest regards for your wellbeing. Be assured that you are not alone in your heart-healthy journey, regardless of how long you have been traveling this path. You are surrounded by a supportive network that is there to encourage you and offer assistance when needed.

We appreciate you including us in your quest for improved cardiac health. The **"Coronary Artery Disease Diet Cookbook for Newly Diagnosed"** is intended to be a helpful tool and traveling partner for you as you pursue a happier, healthier lifestyle.